The
YOGA LIFE

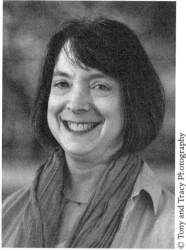

About Ilene S. Rosen

Ilene Rosen, M.Ed, C-IAYT, has been an educator, writer, and yoga practitioner for more than twenty-five years. More recently, she became a registered yoga instructor for adults and children, and completed the YogaLife Institute program with Bob Butera to become a certified yoga therapist. Ilene currently owns InsightEd Educational Consulting company, where she applies her knowledge of yoga, education, and writing to help students and families with emotional challenges navigate the transition from high school to higher education. InsightEdEC.com.

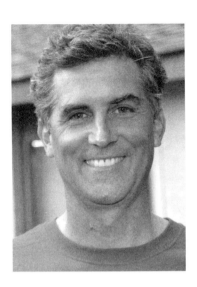

About Robert Butera, PhD

Robert Butera, M.Div., Ph.D., directs YogaLife Institute presently in an online format to train Yoga and Meditation Teachers and Yoga Therapists. He published *Yoga Living* magazine for twenty years. The Yoga programs follow Bob's books, *The Pure Heart of Yoga: 10 Essential Steps to Transformation* (Llewellyn, 2009), *Meditation for Your Life: Creating a Plan That Suits Your Style* (Llewellyn, 2012), *Yoga Therapy for Stress and Anxiety: Create a Personalized Holistic Plan to Balance Your Life* (Llewellyn, 2015), *Llewellyn's Complete Book of Mindful Living: Awareness & Meditation Practices for Living in the Present Moment* (Llewellyn, 2016), and *Body Mindful: Create a Powerful and Affirming Relationship with Your Body* (Llewellyn, 2018). Visit him online at www.YogaLifeInstitute.com.

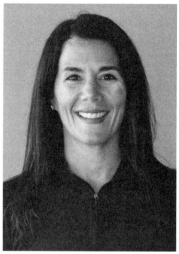

About Jennifer Hilbert

Jennifer Hilbert, MSc., CYT, has been in scientific research for twenty years, where she has worked in drug research in a lab, clinical research, and consulting. She has a Master's degree in Neuroscience with a concentration in Immunology. She has practiced yoga as a teenager and went on to take a 200-hour yoga teacher training in 2011 and a three year comprehensive Yoga Therapy training, both at YogaLife Institute. Jennifer teaches many styles of yoga classes from fitness to healing Yin Yoga. She teaches Physiology and Yoga Therapy seminars. Nutritional instruction and health food cuisine are also strong passions of hers.

The
YOGA LIFE

applying
comprehensive yoga therapy
to all areas of your life

ILENE S. ROSEN

ROBERT BUTERA, PHD · JENNIFER HILBERT, MS

Llewellyn Publications
Woodbury, Minnesota

FIRST EDITION
First Printing, 2021

Book design by Samantha Peterson
Cover design by Shira Atakpu
Editing by Laura Kurtz
Koshas figure by Llewellyn Art Department

Llewellyn Publications is a registered trademark of Llewellyn Worldwide Ltd.

Library of Congress Cataloging-in-Publication Data
Names: Butera, Robert, author. | Rosen, Ilene S., author. | Hilbert,
    Jennifer, author.
Title: The yoga life : applying comprehensive yoga therapy to all areas of
    your life / Robert Butera, PhD, Ilene S. Rosen, Jennifer Hilbert.
Description: First edition. | Woodbury, Minnesota : Llewellyn Publications,
    2021. | Includes bibliographical references. | Summary: "About how the
    branches of yoga may be applied to areas of life through an
    individualized program that best fits the individual's body's need and
    lifestyle. Examines yoga's philosophy and guiding principles, with both
    scientific and philosophical wisdom"— Provided by publisher.
Identifiers: LCCN 2021008645 (print) | LCCN 2021008646 (ebook) | ISBN
    9780738757674 (paperback) | ISBN 9780738757902 (ebook)
Subjects: LCSH: Yoga.
Classification: LCC B132.Y6 B88 2021 (print) | LCC B132.Y6 (ebook) | DDC
    294.5/436—dc23
LC record available at https://lccn.loc.gov/2021008645
LC ebook record available at https://lccn.loc.gov/2021008646

Llewellyn Worldwide Ltd. does not participate in, endorse, or have any authority or responsibility concerning private business transactions between our authors and the public.
   All mail addressed to the author is forwarded but the publisher cannot, unless specifically instructed by the author, give out an address or phone number.
   Any internet references contained in this work are current at publication time, but the publisher cannot guarantee that a specific location will continue to be maintained. Please refer to the publisher's website for links to authors' websites and other sources.

Llewellyn Publications
A Division of Llewellyn Worldwide Ltd.
2143 Wooddale Drive
Woodbury, MN 55125-2989
www.llewellyn.com

Printed in the United States of America

Other Books by Robert Butera, PhD

*The Pure Heart of Yoga, 10 Steps to
Transformation* (Llewellyn, 2009)

*Meditation for Your Life: Creating a Plan
That Suits Your Style* (Llewellyn, 2012)

*Yoga Therapy for Stress and Anxiety: Create a Personalized
Holistic Plan to Balance Your Life* (Llewellyn, 2015)

*Body Mindful: Create a Powerful and Affirming
Relationship with Your Body* (Llewellyn, 2018)

Other Books by Ilene S. Rosen

*Yoga and Mindfulness for Young Children: Poses for Play, Learning,
and Peace* by Maureen Heil and Ilene S. Rosen (Redleaf Press, 2020)

Dedication

This book is dedicated to the yoga community at large and honors the work that has been done to adapt the teachings of yoga to modern life in the form of yoga therapy. As a result of all of your efforts, people from all walks of life have discovered that continued yoga practice and study has the potential to bring out the best in humanity. Thank you for your efforts to make the world a better place.

CONTENTS

PART FOUR: INTRAPERSONAL HEALTH 171

EXERCISES

DISCLAIMER

The practices, movements, and methods described in this book should not be used as an alternative to professional diagnosis or treatment. The authors and publisher of this book are not responsible in any manner whatsoever for any injury or negative effects that might occur through following the instructions and advice contained in this book. Before beginning any treatment or exercise program, it is recommended that you consult medical professionals to determine whether you should undertake the course of practice.

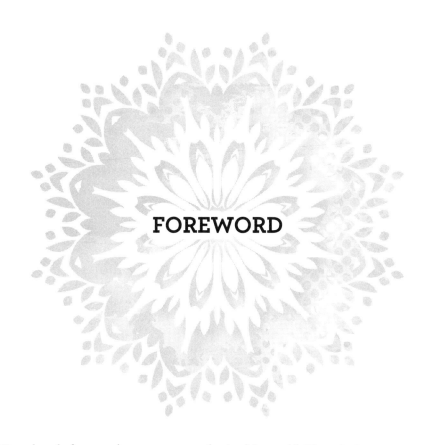

FOREWORD

You already know who you want to be in this world. Yoga, in its pure sense, connects the person we think we are to the person we truly are. This is true for all of us, whether we practice yoga or not. Each of us has a vision of ourselves that we strive toward. Some days we are better at aligning with that self than others. Follow the Comprehensive Yoga therapy model in this book to build days of contentment, well-being, and confidence. Part of the framework you will read about deconstructs the barriers in systematic and stress-free ways. The yoga education here helps us do that by providing a formula to examine the obstacles that stand between us and our vision of ourselves.

Many people suffer from traumatic experiences, anxiety, depression, lack of confidence, issues with food and body image, as well as physical ailments, chronic and acute disease, and pain. Yoga is being established as a useful part of recovery. As readers customize their journey through this book, they have the opportunity to build a life of ease. Through the education and exercises you'll find here, troubling symptoms and habits transform. There are innumerable opportunities contained in this book, available to a range of readers.

The Yoga Life is an excellent resource to support you in your process of becoming. It only takes a few specific, simple changes to feel much better. Life, and our thoughts and beliefs about life, align with harmony and confidence. There's an improvement in your sense of self. Health and well-being bring a flow of joy. This approach provides a road map through clear, actionable steps to create a balanced life. You are the one who decides what this life looks like—it's yours! The beauty of this book is that it guides you with clear explanations and activities.

As you continue to revisit and work with this book, enjoy the process of selecting your goals in multiple realms of life. Since we cannot separate ourselves into bits and pieces—what we do in one area affects the whole— believe in your choices. I find it helpful to remember that any effort toward self-improvement creates ripples of improvement in all areas. For example, a person who simply focuses on hydration may also enjoy improved sleep, increased mindfulness, and greater ease in social situations. All because of one little change. I am excited for the myriad possibilities afforded to readers; they create ripples of improvement. When we acknowledge and accept our habits, automatic reactions, gifts, interests, weaknesses, and heartfelt intentions, we can sculpt our lives into the shape that uniquely suits us. Comprehensive Yoga therapy simplifies this process, making it accessible to all kinds of people. Long-term practitioners, yoga therapists, professionals seeking new ways of supporting clients, and folks who have never even tried yoga can all benefit from this book!

One of the most exciting aspects of Comprehensive Yoga therapy is the opportunity it brings us to comprehend the truths of ourselves. We are so deep and rich; there is much to discover within each of us. As we become more aware of what stops us from living into that vision of ourselves—those beliefs and automatic reactions—the more opportunity we have to stop unhealthy patterns before they ramp up. Thus, we deepen self-understanding and compassion. We are empowered to intervene in our own lives, get rid of negative thoughts and self-harming choices, and direct ourselves back toward what is most important … whatever that may be for you. You define your own priority.

It's been more than twenty years since I needed an academic advisor holding an accredited PhD in yoga therapy. Robert "Bob" Butera fit the description and, lucky for me, accepted my request. We have been collaborating in the field of yoga therapy ever since. I was truly honored and pleased when he asked me to write the foreword for this outstanding book. It was in Comprehensive Yoga therapist training that I had the pleasure of working with both Ilene Rosen and Jennifer Hilbert. It's been a genuine honor to witness each of them continuing to grow and make contributions to the field of yoga therapy, including this stellar book.

Each of these authors approach yoga therapy in a manner that addresses the whole person, and that finesse is evident in this book. People seek yoga therapy for many different reasons. It could be for stress management, or to understand the nuance of enlightenment. Maybe the intention is to establish daily meditation or maybe it's recovery from other physical, psychological, emotional, or spiritual issues. Comprehensive Yoga therapy is a lifestyle-based program. This way, readers make concrete and lasting changes for life. The reasons people seek yoga therapy are as diverse as each of us. A customized lifestyle plan is inclusive and compelling. Each page is targeted toward helping readers create personally meaningful shifts. Through taking those small, significant steps, life is improved day by day, week by week, year by year. This book offers tools, philosophy, and concrete steps to propel you in the direction of your dreams.

May you enjoy the calm, hopeful inspiration of Comprehensive Yoga therapy. Wishing you smiles as you witness the multitude of expected and unanticipated benefits of using this great book.

Erin Byron, MA, E-RYT500, C-IAYT
Registered Psychotherapist
Comprehensive Yoga Therapist
Brantford, Ontario, Canada
December 3, 2019

INTRODUCTION

Comprehensive Yoga therapy is holistic lifestyle education derived from classical yoga that restores balance to our physical, mental, emotional, and spiritual health. It is a system that teaches us how to compassionately evaluate the beautiful intricacy of our whole being and identify how to remove obstacles to health. This holistic perspective upholds that all parts of a human being share equal importance. Scientific and medical perspectives have demonstrated the benefits of understanding a body part or system independent of the whole. Using both models together—holistic and scientific/medical—expands the realm of potential for our health by drawing on the wisdom of ancient practices and modern innovations. In this way, Comprehensive Yoga therapy works in conjunction with medical and allopathic approaches to healing and advocates for holistic modalities such as naturopathy, chiropractic, osteopathy, Ayurveda, and psychological counseling. It is based on the guidance of ancient yogic texts, specifically the *Yoga Sutras,* the *Upanishads,* and the *Bhagavad Gita,* in addition to modern medical discoveries.

What Is Comprehensive Yoga Therapy?

Yoga therapy is different from other kinds of therapy, which aim to treat the symptoms of diseases, and it is also dissimilar to yoga classes, wherein participants follow a sequence of poses led by the teacher. The word *yoga* means "unity," and yoga poses are one part of this unification process. According to the *Yoga Sutras*, one of the primary texts of yoga, "Yoga is the stilling of the waves of the mind" (chapter 1: 2). In popular Western culture, yoga is considered to be movements or postures to increase strength and flexibility; however, the original intention of these postures was to create inner steadiness and comfort for the purpose of transcending all dis-ease and uniting with pure consciousness (*Yoga Sutras*, chapter 2: 46–48). Postures are applied in conjunction with ethical and moral principles, breathing exercises, mastery of sensory stimulation, mental focus, meditation, and connection to a state of pure peace. When such a comprehensive plan is followed, people report greater health, not just in their bodies but also in relationships, emotions, thoughts, and overall sense of connection to goodness in their lives. In the chapters that follow, you will learn how to apply the whole system of yoga to each area of your life.

Yoga therapy is a highly personalized and therapeutic experience focused on the client's goals. When done in a private session with the guidance of a certified yoga therapist, clients explore various elements of the entire system of yoga. Depending on the client's goals and preferences, yoga therapy sessions include a mixture of discussion, education on lifestyle, yoga philosophy and direct experiences, yoga poses, breathing exercises, guided relaxation, meditation, and grounding methods. Common goals for individuals seeking yoga therapy include but are not limited to lifestyle changes; optimal health; disease management; eliminating or managing stress, pain, and emotional distress; mental health, and spiritual growth. The exercises in the opening chapters of *The Yoga Life* will help you clarify your health goals and guide you through an individualized approach to realizing your personal, unique goals.

The field of yoga therapy is increasingly recognized as a scientifically valid approach to physical and mental health. More and more, medical and mental health physicians are referring clients to yoga classes and yoga therapy for a variety of reasons, most commonly to manage stress, anxiety, and pain. Breathing exercises can help calm anxiety, slow down spinning thinking, and cultivate presence and mental clarity. Yoga poses build mental and physical strength and can help lead to more comfort in and appreciation for one's bodies. The movements can also be rehabilitating, easing, and healing for pain. Improvement in mood and self-esteem often occur as the yoga practices developed in session are carried into daily life, creating a sense of personal empowerment in one's wellness. The core yoga philosophies of kindness, compassion, and acceptance (to name just a few) are extremely valuable for reframing self-limiting beliefs.

As an integrative system of amplifying and restoring health, the Comprehensive Yoga therapy process educates about how to make clinically proven healthful choices about work, nutrition, rest, relationships, movement, and thoughts. Healthful choices combined with the balancing nature of yoga practices can reduce stress and internal inflammation, slow physical degeneration, amplify the immune response, help regulate gland and organ functions, clear and balance the vital energy, and increase range of motion and pain-free mobility.

The principles and practices of Comprehensive Yoga therapy described in this book teach a non-prescriptive, unifying approach to health. They also offer a lens through which to view yourself as a whole human being with unique qualities, each one contributing to your overall health in meaningful ways. By considering lifestyle, personality, history, and the mind-body relationship, Comprehensive Yoga therapy expands the definition of health to encompass a whole-person point of view. This means all areas of your life contribute to your health. Did you know your attitudes about finances, work, and relaxation contribute to your health? Or that laughter and hobbies are just as important to include in your daily life as is movement and a wholesome diet? It's true!

Exploring your own health with this whole-person approach will help you integrate a more comprehensive approach to wellness. This book highlights how the field of yoga connects each part of a human being in a context of the other. In other words, you can't study one system of the body or aspect of your life without learning from the others. Comprehensive Yoga therapy is designed to help you cultivate health and harmony in all areas of your life.

Ultimately, yoga teaches us to seek inward, for inside resides the answers to how to live our fullest, most vital life. *The Yoga Life* empowers you to compassionately evaluate the beautiful intricacy of your whole being and identify how to remove obstacles to health, so that you can cultivate more vitality to support your physical, emotional, mental, and spiritual wellness.

Comprehensive Yoga therapy offers a foundation upon which you may reclaim your health and attend to your whole self. This includes being proactive or empowered to take control of the lifestyle factors that predispose you to ailments. It also includes being participatory or engaged in effecting positive change in all areas of your life. And finally, the program is personalized, allowing you to view yourself as an individual and receive personally meaningful tools designed to support your physical, mental, intellectual, and spiritual health. Each of these points emphasize the personal power you hold to create health in all areas of your life, and our book is designed to support you along the way.

Who Is It For?

Comprehensive Yoga therapy is accessible to all people, no matter their age, weight, or abilities. This modality supports our physical body, energy, senses, intellect, and spirit with movements, breathing exercises, mental techniques, lifestyle education, and personal growth philosophy, bringing physical and psychological processes into balance and restoring vitality throughout our whole system.

It should be noted that Comprehensive Yoga therapy and the yoga therapists certified in it to work with clients is not designed to diagnose disease or treat with the intention of making a disease or condition go away. Instead, Comprehensive Yoga therapy will help you significantly improve your quality of life due to the practical application of yoga as it relates to your unique life situation.

As you embark on your yoga therapy journey, continue working with your care providers and seek help as it would benefit you. If you have chronic depression, anxiety, or physical health issues, please be sure to consult with professionals. Should you wish to connect with a Comprehensive Yoga therapist, you may find more information at www.YogaLifeInstitute.com.

How to Use This Book

In each chapter, please read the recommended exercises as thought-provoking applications of the material being introduced. Some readers enjoy writing out notes from the exercises; this is not required, however. You may wish to read through the book and revisit any areas of higher need or interest. Please know that the exercises are helpful integration tools and are intended to educate.

We start with you, as a person, and how you live your life. That is how we have been successful in guiding yoga therapy clients toward better health, and it is the approach we take in this book. You will find here many references to scientific and medical information. These are based on research studies from various fields and provide valuable information. If research on any of the lifestyle topics in this book interests you, we encourage you to explore it further. The bibliography provides a starting point.

Yoga therapy is highly individualized. As yoga therapists, we treat our clients as the individuals they are, with unique DNA, outlooks, concerns, and circumstances that determine what works for them on a practical basis and what is best for their individual health. One way to think of yoga is as a technology for reducing stress and increasing vitality. Comprehensive Yoga therapy looks at each human being as a whole, complete person, then assesses the lifestyle choices that add to or steal from health, and finally works to support the positive aspects while creating real, lasting change. Therefore, this book will not prescribe a specific diet or exercise program to follow, or recommend a certain number of minutes per day you should meditate. Instead, we offer tons of information for you to contemplate along with personal examples and questions designed to inspire you, so you can begin to make changes in your own life.

Each chapter relates to a different aspect of living our health. All areas of life, including exercise, nutrition, sleep, work, relationships, environment, finances, recreation, meditation and spirituality, are opportunities to improve ourselves. Our intention is to encourage and support you to consider your lifestyle and think about where you can make improvements and what changes you are ready to make, to bring yourself closer to comprehensive health.

Steps to Personal Transformation

The book highlights four steps to take toward lasting, positive change, beginning with honest self-evaluation through Listening.[1] After understanding a starting position, then the student is ready for Learning. Practice takes time as you learn to Love the process and later Live it by teaching or demonstrating the new behavior. You'll see each of these four steps come up as we delve into the various lifestyle categories throughout the book.

- Step 1: Listen to know your starting point

- Step 2: Learn new material

- Step 3: Love healthy patterns by practicing new behaviors on your own

- Step 4: Live by integrating new attitudes into your daily interactions

•••• ● ••••

This book sees each area of life to be of vital importance and inherently capable in the process of strengthening our overall health. The motive we bring to any activity can transform it into a health-promoting experience. Let's begin.

---

1. These four steps are part of the Butera Method of Personal Transformation.

part one
FOUNDATIONS

The chapters in part 1 expand the definition of yoga from the realm of fitness classes to holistic lifestyle awareness. If you are already a yoga practitioner, you will meet a broader definition of practicing as an overall system of health. If you are new to yoga, you may be surprised how many healthy living behaviors you already practice. Western perspectives will be connected to Eastern perspectives through various lifestyle reflection exercises. As you progress through the exercises, you will see how each area of your life working in harmony can create synergistic changes that ripple out into all areas of your life.

one
COMPREHENSIVE YOGA THERAPY

Yoga's growth and increasing respect in our society has helped create a landscape rich with options for "doing" yoga. Without a doubt, it is great that so many people are gaining health benefits when they move, stretch, and maybe sweat when they go to a class and do yoga poses. But what about the rest of the day? How can we use the full range of yoga—that is, the complete lifestyle system of yoga that includes so much more than poses—to support our health both on and off the mat?

Despite the popular understanding of yoga as poses or a workout, there are worlds more to it—an abundance of possibilities to practice yoga every day and anywhere to support all aspects of our health. Take away the workout aspects of yoga and you find a beautiful, rich, old, wise tradition and history designed to help us achieve whole-person health. It is these gems of wisdom, originating in ancient India and passed from teacher to student across generations and continents, that will shape your journey throughout this book.

The History of the "Householder Yogi"

At its heart, this book teaches a beautiful history and lineage between nations and teachers, a story rich in the classical Yoga heritage that informs Comprehensive Yoga therapy. With each page you read and yoga practice you do in this book, you, too, become part of this special lineage, thereby connecting you to a network of yoga practitioners throughout the ages and all over the world.

Shri Yogendra founded The Yoga Institute in Santacruz, Mumbai, India, in 1918. The Yoga Institute was the first yoga center in the world open to the general public. As a young college student, Shri Yogendra became an ardent believer in Yoga when he met his guru Paramahamsa Madhavadasaj. Shri Yogendra followed a different course than most of the students of his day. An only son, he had promised his widowed father he would marry and become a "householder" rather than remain a celibate yogi. This promise paved the way for Shri Yogendra to spearhead the movement known as "Yoga for the Householder." This decision was revolutionary in the Yoga world, as up until that point, Yoga was traditionally taught only to an inner circle of gurus in monastic settings without wives and children.

Shri Yogendra believed that many people came to Yoga searching for solutions to their health problems. He committed his life to teaching, researching, and writing about how removing obstacles to health with Yoga would gradually lead people to a better way of living.

Shri Yogendra passed away in 1989. His eldest son, Dr. Jayadeva Yogendra, took over directorship of The Yoga Institute in 1985 and continued his father's teaching until passing away in 2018. Dr. Jayadeva Yogendra introduced several new courses and pioneered work in Yoga Education and Therapeutics. He also authored several books on Yoga education and was the editor of the *Yoga Institute* magazine, which is distributed worldwide. His wife and present director of the institute, Smt. Hansaji, is a well-known speaker who is celebrated for her vibrant and lively talks. Her simple and practical approach to Yoga as a way of life continues to spread the teachings of classical Yoga as a wellspring for health.

The Legacy and Lineage Continues

In 1989, Robert Butera, PhD, one of the authors of this book, trained daily at The Yoga Institute of Mumbai with Dr. Jayadeva Yogendra. Bob lived at the Institute for six months doing intensive personal applications of Yoga philosophy along with Classical Yoga and Yoga Therapy Teacher Training. He taught Yoga while he was in India, and upon returning home he began teaching Classical Yoga philosophy and practices in the United States, opening YogaLife Institute in Pennsylvania in 1996. During this time, he also completed a PhD dissertation, *A Comprehensive Yoga Lifestyle Program for People Living with HIV/AIDS*. The program was modeled after the holistic programs from The Yoga Institute.

YogaLife Institute is the North American Headquarters of the 100 Yoga Centers program sponsored by The Yoga Institute of Mumbai, India. While the main branch of The Yoga Institute is in India, like the YogaLife Institute in the United States, there are other centers inspired by The Yoga Institute's approach in Australia, Brazil, Canada, Finland, Spain, France, Italy, Switzerland, Hong Kong, Thailand, the United Kingdom, and many other countries around the world. Together they all work to carry on Shri Yogendra's vision of bringing the practical applications of classical Yoga philosophy and lifestyle practices into the hearts and minds of householders all over the world, guiding aspirants to acquire "a healthy body, a superior mind, and higher spiritual consciousness."

Embarking on Your Comprehensive Yoga Lifestyle

What is a "yoga lifestyle"? Going to yoga class, drinking green smoothies, and eating a special diet are usually what comes to mind in response to this question. Depending on your preferences and learning style, these answers may be true, but they only tell part of the story of what it means to live a yoga lifestyle. And realistically speaking, you do not even have to do any of those specific things to be living a yoga lifestyle. For example, you may prefer to do your yoga pose practice at home instead of going to a public class. Your digestive system might not like green smoothies, and your body may function most optimally with the diet native to your country. That's totally OK! As you will soon experience, yoga is about tuning in to your own body's needs and wisdom. Learning to pay attention and attend to those needs is just as much yoga as is balancing in Tree Pose.

We invite you to let go of your perceptions of and expectations about what yoga is, what it looks like, who does it, and how it is done. There's no ideal or a one-size-fits all approach. Yoga is for everyone, everywhere, all the time … yes, even for you right now.

In the context of a lifestyle, yoga encompasses an entire system of living, from ancient teachings and philosophies to poses, breathing exercises, meditation, self-study, and more. Ultimately, the pure intention of yoga is self-realization, which means to know oneself. Yoga practices help us to integrate our body, senses, and mind. We can realize obstacles to health and gain clarity about what steps we need to take to help restore balance in our body and life. The repetition of doing these practices can help clear mental clutter and put us in touch with the wisdom of our bodies, from which we can realize our full potential. As we integrate these practices into our daily life, we form a new habit or pattern that ties in directly with brain health. So not only are we doing something beneficial for our bodies, we are literally changing our brains for the better.

A Total Brain Changer

Advances in neuroscience assure us that change is entirely possible. In fact, we can program our brains to help us change. Scientists have known for a long time that children's brains undergo tremendous changes as they grow and learn, a trait called plasticity. But until recently, it was thought that once people reached adulthood, their brains were for the most part fixed with little ability to change. An injury or illness could cause damage to an adult's brain, but otherwise it was believed that not much change occurred.

Now we know that simply isn't true. Using advanced technology called functional magnetic resonance imaging (fMRI) that allows researchers to create images of the brain as it works, we now know that adult brains are also adaptive. New learning, new behavior, and even new *thoughts* create physical changes in the brain. A principal study that led to this conclusion was conducted, perhaps surprisingly, on London cab drivers. Licensed London cabbies are required to pass a famously difficult test showing that they know all the ancient city's roads, businesses, and landmarks. Researchers used fMRI, or functional magnetic resonance imaging, to look at the brains of the drivers, specifically the hippocampus, the area associated with navigation. The drivers' hippocampal regions were larger than average. Researchers believe the change is a direct result of their occupation. When we learn something, our brain creates a new pathway of cells. When we repeat that behavior or that thought, the path becomes stronger, so much so that in some cases researchers can see physical changes in the affected areas of the brain.

A version of this process happens every time we form a new habit. Imagine that you usually take the elevator to your third-floor office, but you want to get more exercise, so you decide to start taking the stairs. You must make a conscious effort to take the new route, and the experience feels new and different. This corresponds to your brain creating a new pathway. Then, the more often you take the stairs, the more familiar it begins to feel. The new feeling is the new pathway getting stronger and stronger in your brain. Eventually the new "stairs" pattern is strong enough that it becomes your default, automatic behavior. You do it without thinking about it. Your brain has created a habit. The old "elevator" pathway is still in there, and you might revert to it at some point, for example if you are very tired or distracted. But it is weaker and more faded. Your brain prefers following the new one.

You can imagine the brain activity like creating a path in the snow: The first time you walk in snow from one point to another, you set down footprints. When you walk that same path repeatedly, the snow becomes packed down and the path becomes clear. It becomes the obvious way to get between those two points.

What does this mean for health? By learning and adopting new, healthier forms of living, you literally change your brain. Your brain, in turn, makes it easier for you to keep up with your lifestyle changes. It takes a bit of work at first to keep from falling back into old habits. In time, the new, healthier habits take on a life of their own.

Yoga Lifestyle Principles and Western Medicine

Comprehensive Yoga therapy that is grounded in the full range of lifestyle factors as outlined in Patanjali's *Yoga Sutras*, the *Bhagavad Gita*, and other ancient yoga texts, in combination with the latest medical research and practices, can help every unique person, just like you, realize health.

The yoga process of self-realization is in many ways the opposite of following a prescription or being a passive patient. The current allopathic, or Western, medical system is limited in the disease treatment process. Although the medical field is gifted at diagnostics and treating some diseases, it lags far behind when it comes to lifestyle support. Research continues to demonstrate how effective lifestyle changes are in combating and preventing chronic disease processes such as heart disease. However, allopathic medicine is not equipped to teach people lifestyle changes. Appointment times are too short, lifestyle research is difficult to conduct, and medical healthcare professionals do not have a complete educational background to deal with the complex issues of lifestyle changes. As a culture, we need to make treating lifestyle-related diseases a priority. It is time for a new way to complement the old, and yoga therapy—a lifestyle approach to health—fills this need.

It should be noted that Comprehensive Yoga therapy (and those certified to work with clients) is not designed to diagnose disease or treat with the intention of making a disease or condition go away. Instead Comprehensive Yoga therapy will help you significantly improve your quality of life due to the practical application of Yoga as it relates to your unique life situation. Nor does yoga therapy prescribe yoga poses to "fix" conditions. Instead, Comprehensive Yoga therapy will help you significantly improve your quality of life due to the practical application of yoga as it relates to your unique life situation. Whether you have picked up this book to address a specific diagnosis or for your general overall health, our aim is to use teachings in Yoga and a variety of practices and exercises to demonstrate how making small changes in every area of your life is the key to physical, mental, and emotional health.

Comprehensive Yoga therapy rests on five equally important fundamental principles These essential and interrelated ideas provide guidance for how to actively engage with your own health.

1. **You are already whole.** Yoga principles embrace a holistic mentality with one guiding precept being that every human being—including you—is already whole, just as you are. You are not broken, and your body is not wrong. Rather, you are whole, and Yoga is a pathway to experiencing your innate wholeness. As you engage with the process laid out in this book, you will realize small steps you can take in your

daily life to enhance your vitality and sense of inner calm throughout your whole, true self.

2. **Every person is unique.** Comprehensive Yoga therapy views each person as a unique individual with unique habits and beliefs that influence their lifestyle. No two people have the same background or lifestyles, and they therefore cannot use the same solutions to solve a problem, especially when it comes to health. For example, an individual reading this book who has low back pain due to an old injury needs different considerations compared to the person reading this book with low back pain due to stress or compared to the person with low back pain due to a difficult relationship at home or at work. In Western health care, the first person might be sent to a physical therapist, the second person to a psychologist, and the third person to a marriage counselor. Comprehensive Yoga therapy applies the principles of Yoga in a practical way, customizing the tools of Yoga for all three of the people with back pain so they can start their healing journey. You can seek out a Comprehensive Yoga therapist to help guide a process uniquely for you.

3. **You are an active student of your own health.** In allopathic medicine the patient's role is to be passively treated for a disease. Yoga takes the opposite approach. We seek to empower you to be a student of your health. The exercises throughout this book seek to help you shine an inward light, examining your body, mind, and spirit, and how they all work together. Learning and understanding your inner self enables you to actively navigate your lifestyle toward greater health, vitality, and wellness.

4. **Healing begins in the mind.** Take yourself in your mind to your favorite place: perhaps a park, the beach, a city you love, or any space that feels peaceful. Reflect on how being in your favorite place affects your thought patterns compared to when you are in a stressful situation. In the former, you are likely more at ease in your body and more present to the moment. In the latter, the stressful situation might set off circular or cyclical thinking and anxiety. Learning how to create calm in our minds is essential to our overall health; as Yoga teaches,

when the mind is calm, the body follows and vice versa. Throughout this book you will learn tools to help calm your mind and find the ease and rest that it needs for deep healing to occur.

5. **Health must be approached from a comprehensive, whole-person point of view to address lifestyle, personality, history, and mind-body relationship.** Allopathic medicine's view of treating by suppressing symptoms of disease processes through pharmaceutical or other physical interventions seldom considers a comprehensive, whole-person point of view. Comprehensive Yoga therapy takes the whole person, the history of the person, and the context of the person into consideration. The athlete has different needs from someone with an illness just as the twenty-something's need differs from an older adult. This framework grounded in yoga allows for deep self-evaluation to identify a problem's root cause, figure out small steps to foster improvement, set goals to practice new habits, and live these new habits that synergistically support your body, mind, and whole health.

Identifying Your Health Intention

As you journey through this book, the lifestyle principles will serve as anchors, keeping you connected to a holistic approach to health grounded in yoga. And as you explore various aspects of your lifestyle (fitness, nourishment, sleep and rest, work, relationships, environment, finance, joy and recreation, relaxation and meditation, and spirituality) in the upcoming chapters, these guiding precepts offer a framework through which to understand the function and purpose of the yoga journey on which you are embarking.

Another powerful anchor is an intention. In yogic philosophy an intention refers to a heartfelt desire, a solemn vow, or a resolve to do something. An intention is a powerful motivational tool for manifesting your heart's desire in your life and health. Sometimes mistaken for goal setting, an intention is the yogic counter to the mindset we often use when embarking on life changes. For example, many of us have experienced the excitement and promise of a New Year's resolution, only to find that by about six to eight weeks in (the national average), we have lost our "will power" and abandon the new behaviors only to return to old habits and patterns. What started off as a promising journey to happiness and possibility leaves us feeling worse off than when we began.

When we view that scenario from a yogic perspective, our resolutions often fail because they are approached from the mindset that there is something wrong with us that needs changing. We set the resolution in the first place because we believe something is inherently flawed within us that is preventing us from experiencing true joy and happiness in our lives. When we shift our approach and come from a place of abundance versus lack, acting from the belief that we already have within us that which is needed to realize our heartfelt desire, we discover that our path is less cluttered. Our journey flows with a renewed sense of purpose and ease. Self-love, acceptance, and joy become accessible, allowing us to realize our most heartfelt desires.

Here are a few examples of intentions one might set for their health:

- My intention is to cultivate joy in my activities.
- My intention is to appreciate all that my body does for me.
- My intention is to connect with my vitality.
- My intention is to cultivate patience with myself as I build strength.
- My intention is to find the courage to try new things.

EXERCISE Setting Your Intention for Your Comprehensive Yoga Therapy Journey

Take a few moments to consider what inspired you to read this book. How did you feel you might benefit from it? When you are ready, use the examples above to help guide you as you set your personal intentions regarding what you wish to receive by going through the lessons and the exercises included here.

Consider the following:

- Use current tense language (*I am* instead of *I will*).
- Keep it short (just a few words).
- Keep it positive (state what you *want* rather than what you *do not want*).
- Make it personal and appropriate to *your* life.

Record your intentions in your journal. If you like, use color to write them out or draw images around them to help anchor them. Imagine how or what you will feel as you embody each of these intentions.

Hold your intentions and the feelings you imagined forward as you continue through this book, referring back to this journal entry regularly.

Chapter Summary

In this chapter, you were asked to let go of the idea that yoga is poses in a class or studio and think of it as a full lifestyle based on a system of teachings and philosophies from ancient India. You learned how adopting new habits can actually change your brain to help you on the way toward greater health. The Comprehensive Yoga therapy approach differs from and complements the Western, allopathic approach to medicine. It follows five main precepts:

1. You are already whole.
2. Every person is unique.
3. You are an active student of your own health.
4. Healing begins in the mind.
5. Health must be approached from a comprehensive, whole-person point of view to address lifestyle, personality, history, and mind-body relationship.

Finally, you set an intention for your health. Remember, this intention can evolve and grow with you.

• • • • ● • • • •

Yoga is a journey of self-realization that helps restore balance in our body and our lives. Through a combination of yoga philosophy, scientific research, personal examples, and introspective questions, this book is designed to inspire you toward improved health and well-being.

In the next chapter, we will begin exploring different paths that yoga offers and the ten lifestyle areas for whole health.

Two

HONORING YOUR
LEARNING STYLE

This chapter aims to move you out of your school desk chair or library seat where you were told to learn by memorizing facts and synthesizing knowledge in a linear fashion for a test. You were told to please the teacher, satisfy the school academic curriculum and eventually fit into a society that is based on creating well-behaved members by repetitive conditioning. Health, therefore, would be more of the same: follow the doctor's orders and you will be fine.

The problem with this one-size-fits-all approach is that the student is stripped of personal power and self-reliance. In this chapter, we invite you to learn how your natural disposition can be your ally when it comes to creating a healthy lifestyle. As you explore the ideas in this chapter, remember that your health plan will be unique to your needs, and the manner with which you carry out this plan is also going to be in your personal style. Let's go for it!

Attuning to Your Inner Wisdom

The health intention you created in chapter 1 is like a seedling preparing to push through the earth and grow according to the natural intelligence encoded in its DNA. You, too, have a natural intelligence called wisdom. Your inner wisdom reveals itself in many forms, including "gut" feelings, thoughts, sensations, hunger, fullness, tiredness, energy, aches, dreams, and much more. Some messages are subtle, others are more obvious. No matter their intensity, these messages serve a purpose: to get your attention because they have something important to communicate.

For example, some people find that a consistent daily routine permits them to feel calm, stable, and directed. In this setting, various personal rituals as simple as a morning cup of tea and some silent meditation can be the best way to listen to one's inner wisdom. However, to the contrary of this regular person is the more emotional personality that thrives in diversity, sometimes staying up late at night, other times seeking inspiration at sunrise. Still others find guidance via relationships and times of prayerful quiet. More physical people enjoy movement and the outdoors as their source of grounding influence. And yet others thrive from studying the big ideas written by great thinkers. These sorts of personalities are discussed later, in "The Paths of Yoga" section of this chapter. Notice elements of each that ring true for you, as we are all a mixture of various personality types.

Learning to first "hear" or trust our wisdom and then respond appropriately is where it can get sticky, when the message relates to making a change in our lives. For example, if I know that a new diet is better for me, I may resist it; or if a new exercise routine is better at this stage of life, I may miss the past activity. Plus, listening to our mind and body is not a skill we are often taught in society, thus doing so in the beginning can feel difficult or even silly, and that's OK. You are not alone in those feelings. The truth is most of us initially come to yoga not in tune with our wisdom, which is partly why we take that first yoga class in the first place; we are searching for something, oftentimes related to our physical, mental, emotional, and/or spiritual health. With time and consistency, yoga practices can help us gain awareness about what we are seeking and the steps we need to take to obtain it.

Steps for Cultivating Health

Decades of teaching yoga and observing others awaken to their own inner wisdom through practices like yoga poses, breathing exercises, meditation, and self-study led to the creation of a four-step framework designed to help you attune to your wisdom in focused, manageable, tangible ways and convert it into actions that support wellness in all areas of your life.

Yoga education teaches us how to address our emotional, spiritual, physical, and intellectual health simultaneously. Rather than taking the traditional Western academic approach of separating disciplines of study, such as psychology, religion, and physiology, Yoga education considers, values, and incorporates each aspect of life. For example, nutritional education considers the food you eat as well as how you eat it, with whom you eat it, and why you eat it. Exercise education includes the obvious physical component but also teaches how and why a person's internal mindset is equally important.

The steps of Yoga education—duty, realized knowledge, nonattachment, and mastery—are derived from a branch of Indian philosophy called *Samkhya*. Duty, or *dharma*, is related to our priorities and roles in life, including responsibilities to self, family and friends, work, society, and all of humanity. Knowledge, or *jnana*, refers to physical, emotional, and spiritual self-awareness. Nonattachment, or *vairagya*, is to view our lives as an objective witness, to live with our struggles but not be defined by them. Mastery, or *ishvara aishvarya*, refers to a humble feeling of achievement, satisfaction, and knowledge that can arise from applying duty, knowledge, and nonattachment to one's life.

From these core philosophies we've outlined steps to help you make meaningful changes that proactively support your health in all areas of life. These four steps will help you attune to your inner wisdom and identify how to convert that wisdom into actions that support your overall health. Here are the steps:

1. **Listen:** Know thyself. Study your strengths and weaknesses to determine where you are in your life and identify what you need your next step to be. Naming a starting point allows you to chart a course for future success.

2. **Learn:** Honor what you know and invite new wisdom. Now that you are clearly aware of your starting point, dive into learning what you need to improve your health.

3. **Love:** Set goals to practice new wisdom and habits in your personal life.

4. **Live:** Share new wisdom with others through example.

The first two steps are reflection-based. In yoga, we call this self-study and it is the process of becoming aware of how our actions, thoughts, words, reactions, patterns, and biases affect our daily experiences and overall health. The last two steps, Love and Live, are practice-based. This means you will learn how to incorporate yoga practices into your daily life that support your health intention.

Think of the four steps as the concrete actions you will take throughout your Comprehensive Yoga therapy journey. These steps will come to life for you in the upcoming chapters as you work through each of the exercises. And keep in mind, these are four steps you can apply to all kinds of situations in your life long after you complete this book to help you to continue to approach your health from a whole-person, synergistic mindset.

The Paths of Yoga

The traditional texts of yoga teach a variety of methods toward self-realization. There is one for those who are psychologically inclined and practice mediation, called *raja*; one for those who follow intellect, *jnana*; one for those who prioritize the body-mind complex, *tantra*; one for those who lean into work, *karma*; and one for those who emphasize love and relationships, *bhakti*.

To put these terms in context, reflect for a moment on your individual preferences, learning style, obligations, and interests. Perhaps you are a thinker or maybe you are more of a feeler, inclined to rely on intuition. Maybe you live from your heart or maybe you are more drawn to quiet reflection and meditation. Or perhaps you are motivated by a sense of duty and service. You can likely track your unique qualities to some or all these different yoga paths. Most of us follow all of these paths at the same time but in varying degrees. Learning how to balance yourself in each of these areas of life is the key to living a yoga lifestyle and achieving health. Let's take a closer look at each of the paths.

Raja

Psychological, understanding the mind

Raja means "king," and this route, the yogic path of psychology, is also known as the royal path or the eightfold path. It is a process of understanding the mind and becoming established in meditation, as taught in Patanjali's *Yoga Sutras*. By following this, you will systematically come to understand the nature of your psychology and gain mastery over your state of mind. The eight-fold path involves having an external ethical code of restraining harmful behaviors and an internal ethical code of observing purity. This path includes yoga practices of postures, breathing, sense mastery techniques, and concentration to help steady the mind so that a practitioner can see clearly into their psychology. Its eight limbs offer a road map to a peaceful lifestyle. Through limiting harm, cultivating serenity, moving enough, breathing deeply, choosing uplifting feelings, and focusing the mind, we are readily able to live a calm, meaningful life.

By having an external ethical code of restraints and an internal ethical code of observances, we become more discerning in how we treat others and, more importantly, our selves. The uplifting attitudes of yoga postures, soothing effects of breathing practices, and sense mastery techniques support us in staying calm and understanding our own minds more deeply. This gives us the ability and commitment to remain aware throughout the day. By upholding focus in everyday life, we begin to shape our thought patterns and brains to respond to life with less worry and feel dignified, empowered, and equipped to face life's challenges.

Ultimately, the raja path of yoga trains the mind to be still and limits its habit of creating stress through overthinking. The removal of stress automatically increases our physical and mental health, which directly improves how we feel in our relationships, at work, and life overall. Less stress also clears the way for us to both become aware of and remove the obstacles in our lives to maintaining a lower stress existence.

Jnana

The highest knowledge, seeing the big picture

The yogic path of the intellect is about more than knowing; it is about experiencing. One of the benefits of yoga is that it gives us a *direct experience—*

a real-time, tangible, embodied experience where we are feeling our bodies in sync with our breath, aware of our thoughts, and connected to the present moment. *Jnana* addresses our beliefs, the foundation upon which all of our decisions are made. In some regard, beliefs are the lenses through which we view reality; paradoxically, these same lenses prevent us from seeing reality for what it is. Beliefs are very much *our* truths, but they are not *the* Truth. Arising from our society, family, education, religion, and experience, beliefs feed our desires and habits. If we deeply hold a version of reality that is a certain way, we will act in accordance with it; it is stressful not to act on the belief because of our limited perception. Over time, repeating these actions based on the same preconceived ideas, we become established in habits, whether or not they truly serve the higher self. The habits arose to serve our desires and belief systems, based on our level of understanding.

The trouble that arises is that except in very rare circumstances, our beliefs do not explain reality correctly. Although there may be facets of truth within our perceptions, there tends to be a heavy amount of bias to accurately reflect reality. When beliefs incorrectly explain any part of reality, we feel dissonance or a disconnection from the higher self, who lives in pure truth. Doubt arises out of that disconnection from truth. For most of us, our treasured beliefs operate below conscious radar. In fact, many self-serving desires—and even some selfless ones—do a good job of keeping themselves hidden.

The good news is that once we see a belief for what it is, we are able to edit it. Beliefs are continually changing, either through conscious effort or through not-conscious processes of integrating learning. Above all, we will always have beliefs; without them, we may become aloof, indecisive, or unproductive. To put it another way, without beliefs we have no foundation. So how can we use them to create a life of well-being rather than stress? We are moving in the direction of realized knowledge, where our beliefs are based on direct experience and higher perspective, not the lowly programming of hopes, expectations, or fears. The yogic path of the intellect teaches that it is important to explore and refine our beliefs and understanding.

There is a vast difference between knowing something intellectually and demonstrating understanding by actually living in alignment with what is known. Realized knowledge arises from the experience of doing something and cannot be taught in any other way.

The hallmark of someone with realized knowledge is a noticeable shift from having information to using it. The person has gone from knowing to doing. Wisdom is reflected in their routines and lifestyle choices, in all the areas where they possess this realized knowledge. Ultimately, the power of realized knowledge supports us in changing our habits and understanding why we really do what we do, and it also offers the perspective needed to let go of stress and anxiety. In a state of realized knowledge, we are able to acknowledge stressful internal chatter without becoming involved with it. The voice of wisdom within us is able to discern between the worried, judgmental lower self and the pure, connected higher self, and it is the latter that we trust.

By recruiting the power of your intellect, you can transcend stress. The yogic path of the intellect reminds us that shifting from *having* information to *using* it will change your life. Living in accordance with your deep, true beliefs and communing with the higher self is uplifting and empowering.

Tantra
Mind-body health, harmonizing energy
Classical Yoga's comprehensive lifestyle approach revitalizes ancient methods in the service of physical, energetic, mental, intellectual, and spiritual health. This is the yogic path of health, or *tantra*.

Before modern medicine came along, we had to rely solely on herbs, food, rest, water, community, and ancient healing practices to maintain health. There was very little chronic stress in the world at that time but life expectancy was short—modern medicine has definitely made a difference! We have better access to food and clean water, and the progress of modern medicine has helped us with various disease conditions. Ironically, the modern world has also brought with it a long life filled with stress and anxiety. It is almost comical that the decrease in ancient practices that didn't allow for a long life came from a time when the quality of life was high and stress was low. Unlike our modern medicine, ancient healing methods are based on creating balance. We can use the approach of these ancient methods to rid ourselves from stress so we can benefit from modern medicine and live long, healthy lives.

Nervous system disorders, heart conditions, chronic pain, digestive diseases, autoimmune conditions, sleep disorders, mental health concerns, and many other issues are associated with or worsened by anxiety and stress. While yoga's goal is not only physical, it does confer distinct, powerful benefits to the body. The sense of ease, peace, and well-being from practicing yoga postures result from a harmonization, revitalization, and balancing of all the systems of the body, most notably the nervous system, the musculoskeletal system, the hormonal system, and the healthy circulation of lymph, blood, oxygen, and life energy. Yoga postures and practices can limit the deleterious effects of stress on health.

Traditional yoga practices are a path to steadiness of mind. By connecting with ultimate concepts and experiencing profound peace, contentment, and acceptance, we learn to hold a connection to the higher self through everyday trials. This higher perspective can be likened to a person standing on an overlook, viewing a busy scene from a distance. There is an awareness of the busyness, its causes and effects, but the viewer is not involved. As we gain a broader perspective, our mental and psychological habits become clear. Through this clarity, we can let go of obstacles to our health and connect to what is more important. The yogic path of health reminds us that we must care for our bodies, attend to our mental wellness, get sufficient rest, and consistently eat nutritious whole foods. These practices help balance our vital life energy.

Karma

The path of action or attitude of work

Perhaps the most challenging aspect of creating a lasting spiritual life is that we have to support ourselves in the material world by going to work. It would be easy to remain in a state of peace if we were able to spend our days completing service projects, communing with nature, doing yoga, and meditating, but that kind of life isn't an option for many of us. In fact, the average American will spend 93,600 or more hours at work during the course of a lifetime. That's a lot of time!

The Yogic Path of Work teaches us that all actions—from washing the dishes to closing million-dollar deals—are spiritual opportunities. When we remember our personal purpose while working, we are uplifted by any task. On the other hand, if we perform the work without the perspective of a higher purpose, we feel burdened and stressed. Yoga philosophy offers a way to approach work that keeps us connected to our spiritual purpose. By following the karma approach to work, we can complete any task with ease and peace of mind, be it at home, at work, or even within ourselves. The steps to this philosophy of work are: acceptance, concentration, excellence, and nonattachment. This approach offers us a process for removing the burden of stress by keeping our internal purpose vital and top-of-mind throughout the process of work.

Acceptance means to cultivate acceptance for the task at hand and to recognize that the task itself is neutral; it's the emotional charge that we bring with us to certain tasks that create frustration, stress, anxiety—all of which lead to other health problems. Our cultural norms and typically self-centered approach to life create internal barriers to acceptance. When we identify those barriers, they can no longer silently sabotage our tranquility. Furthermore, as we cultivate awareness of our mental habits, we begin to notice that our initial reactions to most daily requirements involve some form of resistance or negativity. Embracing the yoga teaching that tasks are neutral can transform stressful habits into equanimity and acceptance.

When our minds are set in neutral acceptance, it is easier to focus on work. Concentration occurs when we focus body and mind on one task without distraction so that work can be a meditation. It is easy to describe concentration but very difficult to achieve. Concentration requires continual effort over a long period of time and needs dedication to stay focused and limit distractions. A special amount of patience is required in the work environment, which offers a multitude of interruptions and distractions.

The trick to mastering concentration is the ability to return to the present moment whenever we are distracted. This is a discipline. Practice can start by simply being present with each breath. It does not matter how many times we get distracted, just stay committed to coming back to the present breath as soon as we notice the mind wander off. It *will* wander off, again and again, for the rest of our lives. That's okay. What's important isn't that it wanders;

what's important is bringing it back. There are many training tools for concentration, such as repeating a silent prayer or mantra, sensing body movements, and proactively eliminating distractions. Adjusting our habits, attitudes, beliefs, and intentions can vastly improve concentration as well.

Excellence is the third precept of the yogic path of work. In this philosophy, excellence can relate to the external product of work but more importantly it relates to *internal* excellence. External excellence is demonstrated by a job well done; internal excellence is a sincere endeavor to do our best. It can take a lifetime to strike a balance between excellence in the mind and external performance. Tipping the balance too much to either side of the equation results in less efficiency. If we are obsessed with maintaining peace of mind at work, we may become lazy or unproductive. If we feel pressured to do a great job, we may sacrifice our health or personal relationships. In the end, both internal peace of mind and a high level of performance are needed to have lasting fulfillment in work.

Remember that there is a difference between excellence and perfectionism! It is impossible to do better than our best. Nothing natural is perfect, except in its own way. The same is true for each of us and the results of our labor. When dedicated to excellence in an endeavor, you feel excellent in the moment. This aligns with the previous precepts of acceptance and concentration. The end result of your labors is not relevant to the *experience* of doing your best; when you offer excellence, you have fully given of yourself. Even more, you feel excellent!

When the concept of excellence is applied to daily life, every task can help improve the body-mind health. Excellence in paying bills is a pleasant attitude of appreciation for the service received. Writing clearly on checks and envelopes are also ways to practice excellence. Washing clothes and dishes well, being polite to strangers in public, and waiting patiently at the traffic light are examples of maintaining an excellent state of mind while performing a simple, everyday action. From this perspective, excellence can encompass everything we do in daily life.

And by practicing nonattachment, we can be at peace in every situation. Since we typically cannot control what happens with our work once it is out of our hands, we do not need to carry around worry about the end results.

This frees up our energy and ultimately cultivates vitality that reaches into all areas of our lives.

The nonattached worker views work as a path of spiritual growth; thus, work becomes a privilege rather than a burden. Every task is an opportunity to learn, grow, and elevate ourselves beyond the attachments of life. The previous three precepts relate to this also: being thankful for work elevates our acceptance; a spiritual attitude helps hold our concentration; and committing to excellence is cleansing for the soul.

The yogic path of work reminds us that the greatest, most sustained rewards are internal. In truth, the only thing we have control over is our internal state and our efforts. When we concentrate on what matters and do our best, we can detach from the rest.

We'll revisit karma yoga in chapter 6, "Transforming Work Stress."

Bhakti

Relationships with others and the divine honoring emotion

Bhakti is the yogic path of relationships. Often referred to as the devotional path, those who relate to this path tend to be caring, emotional, sensitive, and attuned to their own as well as others' feelings.

Yoga therapy is effective in helping people manage the emotional nature of relationships. Emotions and health are linked—the Psychosomatic Reality. An upset stomach commonly relates to worry, which binds the vagus nerve complex that links the brain and guts. A heavy heart brings the shoulders forward in times of sadness leading to shortness of breath, back pain, and possibly chest pain. Irritants that we name "a pain in the neck" indicate an underlying psychological state of imbalance. Unlike acute medical pains and diseases, psychosomatic imbalances tend to appear in more subtle or changing ways. However, what begins as subtle levels of stress in the body and mind may lead to anxiety, hypertension, and other health conditions. Yoga therapy helps balance emotions, health, and relationships.

Compared to the vast amount of research on physical ailments, little has been proven about the physical effects of psychosomatic illnesses. However, any person knows that strong, uncomfortable emotional states such as sadness, anger, and worry can lead to mental health issues. This may be true in subtle ways, as well. The effects of strong emotional states on physical health have only been formally researched in recent years, but much has been proven or at least suggested during the short time that this kind of research has been conducted.

Among the most solid research findings are depression's impact on physical health and wellness. Depression slows down our ability to heal from physical illness. Close emotional and social connections tend to lead to longer and healthier lives, while suppressed emotions and lack of closeness tends to lead to a suppressed immune system and increased mortality. So research is finally catching up to something we have always known, our relationships are important for our health.

According to classical Yoga philosophy, the primary purpose in life is to connect to the higher self (which we can interpret as being our healthiest, most vital selves possible, no matter the circumstances). This colors our responsibilities to loved ones, work, and society. Neglecting the fundamental duty of spiritual self-care leads to stress and anxiety. Some typical examples of this personal neglect are over-working, eating poorly, not resting sufficiently, not exercising enough, or emotionally neglecting our families. When we integrate the fundamental purpose of connecting to our higher selves, we are able to restrain impulses, regulate desires, accept internal authority, and commune with our true, calm nature. By prioritizing this elevated state of mind, our relationship stresses diminish. Ultimately, staying true to our fundamental purpose saves us from the internal pain and suffering that inevitably affects our relationships.

Our primary adult relationship begins within our own minds. If we are not perfect at listening to others, it is unlikely that we are listening to our own thoughts and feelings. Self-talk is usually synonymous with self-criticism. We often hear, "I am my own worst critic." Yoga's goal is to flip that around so that we can say, "I am my own best friend! I listen to my ideas, my feelings, and my dreams." We are always talking to ourselves, whether conscious of it or not. It is worth listening to what our thoughts are saying and cultivating uplifting internal messages. It is also important to listen deeply, tuning in to the subtle messages of fatigue, hunger, enthusiasm, and affinity that may be expressed at any given moment. Ultimately, this deep listening hones our innate knowing and makes us better listeners to our loved ones.

The bhakti path of yoga teaches us how to be in balance with our emotions and relationships by prioritizing caring for our higher selves and learning to practice compassion toward others. Living in a state of emotional balance will ripple outward to other areas of our life, aiding in increasing overall health.

Depending on your personality, background, preferences, beliefs, and life experiences, you likely related more strongly to some of the five paths than others. From a traditional yoga standpoint, each one represents a pathway to self-realization, allowing for individual aptitudes, learning styles, obligations and interests to be honored in that process. Not all people practice yoga in the same way, yet all people will benefit from some form of practice, be it dominantly characterized by devotion, meditation, physical poses, selfless service, or intellect.

Using the Yoga Paths for Whole-Person Health

When it comes to cultivating health, the five different paths provide a very useful framework for how to live a yoga lifestyle. We can think of each path as representing a category of lifestyle factors. By focusing on all five paths or lifestyle categories, you strengthen all areas of your life, bringing balance into your physical, mental, emotional, and spiritual health. Compared to medical approaches, which generally seek out one solution to improve a singular aspect of health at a time, when we attend to all the paths of yoga, the entirety of our beings is cared for. Thus seeking small, steady changes in every area of our life is the key to health.

Let's look at these five paths more specifically through the lens of lifestyle categories.

- Raja, or meditation and psychology, relates to self-understanding. We need to devote time to self-understanding so that we can thrive rather than simply survive. Without knowing ourselves, we spin our wheels, oftentimes staying stuck in relationships, jobs, and behaviors that undermine our health. Lifestyle habits that deepen our self-understanding are relaxation and meditation.

- Jnana, the intellect, relates to wisdom put into action and our ability to see the bigger picture. This includes appreciating the value in things like respecting the environment as well as taking time for joy and recreation.

- Tantra, the path of health, relates to the body-mind complex. Lifestyle habits related to physical fitness, nourishment, sleep, and rest come into play here. Removing obstacles to our physical and mental health and then maintaining new health-nurturing habits is the key to this lifestyle category.

- Karma relates to attitudes and beliefs about work and finances. Learning to let go of attachment to outcomes is a lifelong practice, and work and finances present the perfect opportunity to pursue a more neutral and accepting mindset, releasing the energy-draining feelings of worry, stress, and angst around work and money, and embracing a spirit of higher purpose in our tasks.

- Bhakti relates to lifestyle habits associated with relationships and spirituality. Strengthening our self-reliance in relationships and embracing support in spiritual communities and/or practices is essential to health in this area of life.

EXERCISE Seeing the Five Paths in Your Life

Notice which elements of the five paths show up in your life. Is one of the paths more "the real you" than others? Each path is equal in value; the approaches honor different attributes that people have. By knowing your natural baseline, you can rely on your gifts and know your innate strengths!

The small steps you take in one lifestyle category will have ripple effects that extend into the other categories. For example, as you improve your sleep, you might feel happier at work or present in your relationships. Or, after a week of consistently doing ten minutes of yoga poses every morning, you might discover that you have more energy or your mood is uplifted. The scenarios are endless, but one thing is for certain: small changes in each area bring significant shifts in the health of all areas of your life.

Chapter Summary

This chapter described four steps that will guide you through the process of integrating new, healthy habits in your life from a whole-person perspective to address emotional, spiritual, physical and intellectual health simultaneously. The steps are as follows:

- Listen
- Learn
- Love
- Live

You also learned about different paths toward self-realization, and how you can apply them to cultivating health in all areas of your life over the upcoming chapters. By focusing on the five paths, you make small changes that help to strengthen all areas of your life through focusing on your whole being. The paths are:

- Raja: Psychology and meditation
- Jnana: Intellect and wisdom
- Tantra: Health, nurturing habits, and the body-mind complex
- Karma: Work
- Bhakti: Relationships and love

Traveling the Paths Your Way

The next ten chapters are devoted to each lifestyle area: fitness, nourishment, sleep and rest, work, relationships, environment, finances, joy and recreation, relaxation and meditation, and spirituality. Using the four steps of Listen, Learn, Love, and Live, we will guide you to evaluating your relationship with each of these lifestyle areas, figure out what steps you need to take to improve health, devise goals to remove obstacles and practice new, healthy habits, and actively live these healthy behaviors in your daily life.

We encourage you to focus on the areas that are calling you, that you know need attention now, and then circle back to those areas that feel less urgent. In other words, travel the five paths your way—tune in to what feels right to address first, and then go from there. Remember, by simply beginning this process, you are doing something positive for your health. Small shifts are the key—you can do small shifts!

part two
BODY HEALTH

The word "holistic" sometimes has a connotation of doing things differently from the mainstream, such as practicing yoga or drinking smoothies because it is culturally hip. The holistic approach found in the following chapters is about interconnectedness and interdependence—a whole-view approach with three dimensions. A line is two dimensional and can give us information about the world. A globe, however, modifies the map into a three-dimensional, life-like sphere.

The three-dimensional model of lifestyle health provided here considers each of the ten lifestyle aspects in this book as interconnected and interdependent with one another. For example, digesting food requires physical movement and rest, while movement requires energy from food and rest, and so forth. Each lifestyle area addressed in this book is interdependent.

Movement is normally described as a set of exercises that are recommended; however, as you will learn in chapter 3, "Creating a Movement-Based Lifestyle," the Comprehensive Yoga therapy approach expands this thinking to embrace an individualized program that best fits your body's need and lifestyle. In a two-dimensional world, chapter 4 would be called "Diet," but our approach shows instead how "Nourishing Your Whole Self" relates to feeding all levels of the human being from the physical to the spiritual. Chapter 5, "Honoring Rest and Sleep" is more than a discussion on how to sleep; the chapter describes the elements of complete rest and relaxation that are interconnected with sleeping well.

Enjoy this section on how to increase vitality and health in your body!

three
CREATING A MOVEMENT-BASED LIFESTYLE

The yogic path of health reminds us that we must care for our bodies, attend to our mental wellness, get enough rest, and consistently eat nutritious whole foods. This chapter focuses on creating a movement-based lifestyle through the lens of resiliency. You will learn the way in which resiliency is related to health, examine your beliefs about exercise, and be guided to identify obstacles to approaching movement from a self-care mindset. The exercises and yoga practices offer opportunities to experience "balanced movement" as well as set some goals to begin integrating new exercise and movement routines into your daily life.

Movement and Resilience: Manifestations of Health

"If life had to be summarized in just one concept, it would be movement. To live is to keep moving. It is a cycle of activity and rest, and even when we are at rest, movement takes place inside of and all around us."[2] This quote raises our awareness of the beautiful reality that movement is a pure expression of life. If life is movement, then being able to live and move with resiliency—to be able to adapt to challenges of all kinds—is a manifestation of health.

Resiliency is our ability to adapt, cope with stress or change, and bounce back from challenging moments and situations. From a Comprehensive Yoga therapy perspective, movement is an opportunity to increase resiliency on the physical, mental, emotional, and spiritual levels. Put another way, when done with awareness of our bodies' potential as well as limitations, movement can improve our ability to respond to life. From carrying groceries to walking down a staircase to going for a swim, resiliency allows our bodies to adapt to the challenge at hand and move skillfully. We build emotional resilience as we learn to let go of expectations about what we want our bodies to do or be and embrace a more accepting, kinder relationship with our bodies in movement.

When we engage our physical bodies in movement, we nourish all the systems of the body, strengthen the nervous system, and take a break from hard mental work, thus giving our minds an opportunity to rest or gain clarity. Emotionally, movement can help take the edge off stress, anxiety, and depression, uplifting our mood. Embracing movement from a mindset of health or self-care can lead to greater connection with self, as well as a community if done in a group, and even connection with a higher source as we deepen our commitment to our personal health and give ourselves permission to value self-care.

Resilience is very different from the typical, more medically focused measures of health (e.g., weight, body mass index, and blood pressure, to name a few)—in fact, it doesn't describe a certain body type or size at all. We can cultivate resilience for the entire duration of the life span and although it may feel different with age, resiliency is not limited by it. For example, yoga exercises may be adapted to different age groups such as senior's yoga and kid's yoga, or to groups such as yoga for athletes or yoga for singers. Yoga exercises can be intensified by challenging breathing patterns or be gentle poses

---

2. Kristen Butera and Staffan Elgelid, *Yoga Therapy: A Personalized Approach for Your Active Lifestyle* (Champaign, IL: Human Kinetics, 2017), 37.

for a prenatal group, for example. The saying, "yoga is for every body" is not just catchy—it is a reality.

If you've associated movement or exercise (depending on your word preference) with external factors such as weight and size or other numerical indicators, we invite you to consider the internally motivated value of resilience to increase your health. Socially, we are trained to believe that external factors dictate the extent of one's health. From the standpoint of general health (not disease or other major conditions), relying on external factors can become a preoccupation that compromises our self-worth and body image. For example, an external motivation might be to lose weight because of the pressure to succeed based on a societal view of the body. However, if the motivation starts from a point of view of loving life and exercise is coupled with a healthy moderate diet that aligns with a vibrant life, then the motivation is internal. This line of thinking may go something like this: "I am not needing to lose weight today, because I am loving myself as I eat right and exercise." There is no reward after the goal is reached, as the reward of feeling self-worth occurs during the process of making healthful choices. Thus, this internalized healthy living expresses a daily routine, not any sort of short-term sacrifice.

We can also think of resilience and movement in terms of the direct relationship between exercise and our bodies' ability to prevent and fight disease and recover from other health conditions, all of which is adaptation (resiliency) in action. Research has extensively proven the positive relationship between movement and health. Incidents of cancer, heart disease, and many other illnesses are lower when people exercise. If research on the topic of exercise and health interests you, we encourage you to explore it further. The pursuit of knowledge also cultivates a kind of intellectual resilience that equips us with information that in turn allows us to adapt in our decision-making or actions that benefit our health. Use the bibliography at the back of this book as a starting point.

What doesn't benefit our health is a sedentary lifestyle, and there are many studies to support this assertion, too. Due to the nature of our modern lifestyle, a lack of movement more than a few times a day is a reality for many. Technology and the continuously evolving forms of convenience that society values result in less movement and more sitting. For our bodies to stay resilient, they need to move.

For people who lived a hundred or more years ago, movement was a requirement of life. Most had to walk or ride horses to get around, and a great many difficult chores were done by hand. There aren't too many of us today who must saw our own wood or churn our own butter. Normal, physical activities such as brisk walking, gardening, cleaning the house, mowing the lawn, and playing with children all count as aerobic activity that strengthens our bodies and increases vitality.[3] Energy begets energy, and the opposite is also true.

While exercising regularly is a necessary routine to cultivate a healthful yoga lifestyle (a matter explored later in this chapter), we need more than a workout a few times a week to counter our mostly sedentary lifestyles. We need more movement in general (in addition to traditional exercise) to keep our bodies resilient and gain health benefits in other areas of our lives. We also need movement in our daily lives now so that we can move well in our older years.

Medical Recommendations and the Comprehensive Yoga Therapy Perspective

Both the World Health Organization[4] and the CDC[5] (U.S. Centers for Disease Control and Prevention) recommend that most adults get 150 minutes of moderate-intensity aerobic physical activity each week, and twice-weekly muscle strengthening; with moderate intensity defined as just about everything you would think of as exercise, from cardio machines to dance. They point out that exercise doesn't have to be something done only at a gym or in a class—lifting groceries or heavy boxes can build strength in the same way as lifting weights. And while many people might assume that exercise would be

---

3. Editors of TIME, "The Science of Exercise: Younger. Smarter. Stronger," *Time* publications, April 2017.

4. World Health Organization, "Physical Activity and Adults: Recommended levels of physical activity for adults aged 18–64 years." www.who.int/dietphysicalactivity/factsheet_adults/en/.

5. Centers for Disease Control and Prevention. "Why Walk? Why Not!" https://www.cdc.gov/physicalactivity/walking/index.htm.

detrimental to the elderly and ill, research is proving that this is not the case. Exercise is for everyone.

Comprehensive Yoga therapy absolutely supports movement for a healthy lifestyle, but it takes a different slant on decisions about what kinds of exercise we should get, and how much. Instead of a one-size-fits-most prescription, yoga therapy answers these questions from an individualized, self-care mindset. One of yoga therapy's criteria is a practical assessment of how we feel energetically on any given day. This concept holds that everything in the world, including people, is considered in terms of its energy, known in Sanskrit as *gunas*. Each of us at any particular time can feel too little energy (*tamasic*), too much (*rajasic*), or a balanced amount (*sattvic*). Too little energy leads us to lethargy. We feel tired and run down, with not much interest in doing what we have to do. We may find that we need to sit or lie down more often than usual. When we are up and moving, we feel like we're dragging ourselves. Too much energy, on the other hand, leads to busyness, but not the good kind. In this state not only are we going about our business actively, it is in a frenetic manner. Internally we feel anxious and on edge. Balanced energy is where we hit the sweet spot. Our minds and bodies are in sync with our responsibilities. Our actions are efficient, our behavior purposeful. We feel energetic and alive.

The goal for exercise is to find activities that lead us to that centered, balanced, just-right state. That means we want to work hard enough, but not too hard; we want to make a solid effort without tipping into true discomfort. If you finish a weightlifting class or play eighteen rounds of golf you aren't used to and then must rest on the couch for hours, you have expended too much energy. You are left in the *tamasic* state. If your exercise is to walk your dog for a mile but then you still feel restless or *rajasic,* you are left with too much. Of course, if you are overweight, injured, or new to exercise, a short dog walk might be just the right thing to start. The yoga therapy view is not the prescriptive approach we expect from medicine. Instead it's highly individualized and intuitive, and it will change along with you and your situation.

Looking at exercise or movement in this way can be empowering. It allows you to make your own choices and feel comfortable doing what's right for you, rather than comparing yourself to your neighbors or following the general recommendations of people who may be expert in a field of exercise—up to writing books or articles that promote a specific program—but who don't know you and your needs personally.

How do we create more movement in our lives that aligns with our energy and leads us to feel more centered, more balanced, healthier? How do we make our bodies more resilient? What are the obstacles that prevent us from following through on what we know to be good for us? There are many components that go into answering these questions, and the areas we will look in the remainder of this chapter include mindset, seeking balanced movement, making room for movement in your life, honoring and challenging your movement preferences, and creating daily routines and rituals to establish healthy movement habits.

Mindset: Self-Care Versus Punishment

The attitude you bring to any activity is as important as the activity itself. Attitude is comprised of self-talk, body language, beliefs, resistances, and biases—yes, it's a lot to unpack for sure! From a Comprehensive Yoga therapy standpoint, becoming aware of these details leads to improved health, because we can actively identify and examine mindset obstacles and replace them with empowering perspectives and actions that cultivate resilience and lead to increased health. We can also identify those aspects that are already contributing to our health and continue to cultivate them in our lives.

Your answers to the following exercise, both felt and verbal, provide abundant feedback about your attitude toward these words. Let's look at your answers through the lens of punishment and self-care, as these concepts and your beliefs about them are key to figuring out the step(s) you need to take to bring more movement into your life. For many, exercise is paired with a fighting mentality. We approach the treadmill, the weights, or the ball like an enemy to be conquered. Trainers and fitness instructors use this kind of combat mindset to motivate their clients and students in class. Combat language permeates fitness marketing materials and social media, and it is ingrained in our social consciousness—we work out to fix, change, and control our bodies, and the punishment mindset is often present as we strive to achieve "no pain, no gain"-type success. For some people, a combat-driven mindset helps to increase motivation to work hard or move fast—almost like we're pretending we really are the primitive human running from the tiger millions of years ago. But we know that fighting is stressful, just like running for your life would be.

Ignoring the very bodies we are exercising is another all-too-common mindset that often results in physical injury. Joints and muscles issue warning signs before they become injured. Feelings of excessive soreness or strain are how our bodies signal to our brains they are not up to what we're asking of them right now. But many exercise mindsets encourage us to disregard that information. The "no pain, no gain" way of thinking glorifies discomfort. The idea of "soldiering through" makes ignoring pain virtuous and admirable. If you were a high school or college athlete, you were likely trained to work out as though the team's win depended on your ability to push yourself through practice, ignoring how you felt. And while that mindset may have been appropriate for your teenage and young adult self, it becomes a different matter in middle age—a fact that can be very hard to accept.

Simply feeling competitive with the people around us or wanting to perform like we did back in the day add to the list of reasons many of us employ metaphoric earplugs when we exercise. We don't want to hear the warnings our bodies are sending. Instead, we feel more comfortable punishing, because it's a habit we've likely been taught and have repeated throughout our lives.

Below are a few examples of fictitious people. See if you recognize traces of yourself in their stories. Use this insight to help you in the self-reflective exercises that follows.

"No pain no gain" is Joe's mantra. He doesn't want to waste his precious exercise time, so he quickly gets his heart rate up and burns calories. He lives on a cycle of pizza and beer binges on the weekend followed by weekday salads and workouts. Upon reflection, Joe shifts his mantra to feeling alive when he exercises, which allows him to ease himself into his peak intensity. He begins to notice that he feels sluggish after his weekly pizza feasts, so he starts to eat more moderately to feel move alive.

Lori's goal is to run a distance race and finish faster than her sister, so she trains every day in spite of slight pains in her ankle. She ends up injured, frustrated, and unable to run anymore. However, the experience brings her to yoga classes. At first, she compares herself to the more limber people in class, just as she had been stuck in a competitive frame of mind with her sister. The yoga teacher mentions the idea of acceptance of one's own body, and over time Lori comes to adopt this mindset as her own. Eventually, she returns to running and forgets about comparing herself to her sister. She accepts her own abilities and limits while enjoying running on nature trails.

EXERCISE Your Exercise/Movement Starting Point

Let's take some time to reflect on your thoughts, beliefs, and emotions about exercise and movement. Find a quiet place and take out a notebook or journal to write out your thoughts and reactions to the following inquiry. (You may also simply reflect as you read.)

As you go through this exercise, allow yourself to be open and curious as you witness your mental, emotional, and physical responses without judgment. Know that wherever you are is okay. This process of listening provides clarity on where you are so you can see where your next steps lie.

First, write the word "exercise" on the page. Notice any thoughts that arise as you consider the word. What does the word "exercise" mean to you? Are there any memories, beliefs, judgments, images, or words that come to mind? Do you have an emotional response? What do you feel in your body? Become aware of any visceral responses, noting where they are in your body and what they feel like. Remember, your visceral response is loaded with wisdom about your relationship to exercise and your body. It deserves as much of your attention as your other responses.

Take time to write about what comes into your awareness as you consider the word "exercise." Allow these to come together to give you a clear reflection of your relationship with it.

Next, write the word "movement" in your journal. Follow your awareness in the same fashion, noticing thoughts, emotions, physical sensations, and so on. Journal about what you notice. You will come back to these for reference as you progress through the other exercises in this chapter.

Your answers to this exercise, both felt and verbal, provide abundant feedback about your attitude toward these words. Consider your answers through the lens of punishment and self-care, as these concepts and your beliefs about them are key to figuring out the step(s) you need to take to bring more movement into your life

Finally, think back over the past week: what sorts of exercises did you participate in, from formal workouts or classes to simple walking and light activity? Can you identify the mindset behind these exercises?

Below are a few examples of fictitious people that may spark aspects of yourself, please chart your own activities and the mindset.

Self-Care

"Self-care" is popularly defined as the practice of taking action to preserve or improve one's own health. What's your personal definition of self-care? What have you heard others say "self-care" means? If you fall in the camp of people who struggle with defining the term, you are not alone. We promise.

We live in a society that holds productivity as one of the highest, if not the highest value. We must always be doing, going, and doing more to be a productive member of society, as well as of our family, community, partnerships—and the list goes on and on. How else are we to prove our worth? If, while growing up, you were modeled that productivity is indicative of self-worth, then recognizing the value of self-care can be difficult, with fears of laziness, failure, and not doing or being enough always lurking in the background.

When done with the intention of self-care, the practices of yoga fortify our health. And for that matter, performing any activity from a mindset of self-care puts health front and center. We make ourselves a priority. In fact, we are especially "productive" when we are practicing self-care, because the actions we are taking are intentional and purposeful. Our efforts are focused, and we can find ease in the activity (even if it is challenging) because we aren't putting ourselves through the mental and emotional stress that accompanies a punishment mindset. This may be summarized by the externalized and internalized dynamics: external is out of our control and internal is by our choice. The outside pressure can make an activity feel like drudgery, while an attitude shift that puts the same activity within our control can bring joy.

Here are examples of externalized attitudes and internalized attitudes:

- The doctor said to do this vs. *I agree with the doctor, and I wish to care for my health.*

- My coach wants me to train to win vs. *I choose to train for the joy of the sport.*
- I want to be like that person vs. *I honor my unique body and mind.*
- I improve myself to achieve X vs. *I improve myself to reach my full potential.*

What might self-care mean in terms of exercise and movement? The possibilities are many, but one that serves as a helpful example and might resonate is related to injury prevention. Learning to honor our bodies' messages is a lifelong process. The more we practice listening and responding (also known as adapting) appropriately, the more resilient our bodies become. Instead of pushing through a twinge or pain (punishment) and ignoring messages, perhaps what is needed is to vary the exercise routine a bit. Repetitive injuries are an extremely common reason why exercisers require physical therapy. Perhaps you need to look at your form or your alignment to determine how to adapt to what your body is feeling. Maybe all your body needs in that moment is brief rest, or perhaps the support of tape or a brace would make a big difference. Fitness professionals are an often-overlooked source of help and information on injury prevention. We must remind ourselves that listening to our bodies' aches and pains is not weak or soft, it's self-care—a practice of attending to our health.

EXERCISE Reframing Your Mindset Around Exercise

Take a look at your responses from the previous exercise. What is your relationship to "exercise" and "movement"? Do you have a positive experience? Do you resonate more with one word over the other? Do you feel resistance to either word?

Based on your past experiences, you may love to exercise, or the idea may invoke some level of resistance or even anxiety about exercise. The language of punishment regarding exercise often plays a part in shaping our mindset about movement and our bodies. Let's take a look at some phases and practice reframing them from "punishment" to "self-care" mindset.

Punishment Mindset	Self-Care Mindset
No pain, no gain.	Listen to your body. Make adjustments where needed.
Soldier through.	
Push yourself again and again. Don't give an inch until the final buzzer sounds.	
Success trains, failure complains.	
Never give up.	
If your mind tells you to stop, you will stop. Train your mind first and enslave your body to it.	
Go, go, go! Keep pushing!	
All we want is to win, win, win!	

What are some other thoughts that hinder you? Do you have beliefs related to age, weight, abilities, or body type? Perhaps you have beliefs about time, energy, or other obligations that keep you from engaging in a regular exercise routine. Write a list in your journal of any limiting thoughts or beliefs about exercise, then follow the same process to reframe them within a more supportive mindset. Keep this in your journal to reflect on as you develop your plan for introducing or expanding your exercise routine. Here are examples of what your results may be:

Punishment Mindset	Self-Care Mindset
No pain, no gain.	Listen to your body. Make adjustments where needed.
Soldier through.	Align your highest aspirations with your health of mind and body.

Punishment Mindset	Self-Care Mindset
Push yourself again and again. Don't give an inch until the final buzzer sounds.	Appreciate each moment of your playing; it is a gift to be able to participate.
Success trains, failure complains.	Keep a positive attitude about yourself and your teammates.
Never give up.	Strive to reach the zone of higher consciousness while playing.
If your mind tells you to stop, you will stop. Train your mind first and enslave your body to it.	Accept your weakness and find balance from your sport.
Go, go, go! Keep pushing!	Enjoy every minute of your game.
All we want is to win, win, and win.	Turn win into a win-win for all by making your goal self-improvement of mind and body the goal for all.

How to Create Balanced Movement in Daily Life

When we speak of balanced movement, we are referring to an awareness of all the ways our bodies can move, particularly our spines, and incorporating activities that allow for all of these movements to be present. One common movement is simply walking, which circulates blood and benefits the legs. Walking up hills and on uneven surfaces stimulates balance. Picking up items and dressing may activate some forward bending. On occasion, there may be a twist if you look from side to side. However, there is very little to no back bending or side bending in our modern lives.

Integrating movement or activities that encourage all ranges of motion helps to keep our bodies nimble, our nervous systems strong, and helps to balance our whole beings. There are other benefits, too, in other areas of our lives that come from routine, balanced movement. You might sleep better, take more care to prepare your meals, be more present at work, and be just generally a kinder person. Balancing our bodies creates balance in our lives.

Let's look at the components of balanced movement: kinds of exercise and the movements of the spine.

Categories of Exercise

There are four categories of exercise: endurance, strength, balance, and mobility. Endurance, also referred to as aerobic or cardio, gets your heart and lungs moving faster, improving their overall function. Strength training makes your bones and muscles stronger, usually by lifting something heavy or doing weight-bearing exercises. Mobility is the range of motion that we have in our joints and our ability to control that range of motion. Balance is the ability to remain upright and steady. Sometimes practiced as ends in and of themselves, for example during yoga and tai chi, mobility and balance are generally simply part and parcel of other types of exercise. Lifting weights and hitting a tennis ball both require balance and mobility, as well as strength and sometimes endurance.

Movements of the Spine

Spinal health is essential to our body's ability to be resilient—to perform the daily functions of life and adapt to new scenarios and situations that challenge our movement. Our spine can be exercised in five directions: flexion (forward folding), extension (back bending), lateral (side bending), upward (reaching to feel length), and rotation (twisting). Making sure to incorporate these movements into our lives every day is key to building resilient bodies and nervous systems.

One of the main benefits of a balanced yoga class is the amount of movement for the spine. The directional moves of the spine—upward, sideways, forward, backward, and twisting—are included with multiple repetitions. In addition, they activate different areas of the spine: a lower body twist and an upper body twist. For seniors or others who are unable to do a regular class, the same effects can be achieved with chair yoga. Remember, people of all activity levels can benefit from yoga poses. If you have tried yoga, you know how this sort of exercise counterbalances the modern sedentary lifestyle.

Strengthening the Nervous System

Engaging in the five types of exercise and the different movements of the spine nourishes the very system of our body that builds resilience: the nervous system. Let's take a moment to review how it works.

The nervous system is divided into the central nervous system (CNS) and the peripheral nervous system (PNS). The CNS includes the brain and spinal cord. The PNS includes the nerves and nerve bundles, called ganglia, that are outside the CNS. The CNS receives information from the PNS and then decides what to do with it.

The autonomic nervous system (ANS) is part of the PNS and is associated with the visceral organs. It regulates heart rate, respiratory rate, digestion, and other essential internal functions. The ANS is further divided into the sympathetic nervous system (SNS) and parasympathetic nervous system (PNS). The SNS controls the "fight, flight, or freeze" responses that the body makes to danger. The PNS controls "rest and digest," the relaxed bodily activities that occur when we are not in danger.

Stress sets off the SNS, or "fight, flight, or freeze" response. This heightened state is characterized by an increase in heart rate, a decrease in peristalsis (digestion), and an increase of blood to the heart, lungs, brain, and spine. The SNS is highly useful for times of crisis because it allows us to respond appropriately to a threatening situation. However, chronic stress and anxiety, as well as sleep deprivation and exercising past a healthy limit, keeps the SNS activated for too long, not allowing the body a chance to heal or recover and leaving us feeling run down and exhausted.

In contrast, the PNS slows the heart and respiratory rates. Activating the PNS improves the body's functioning, ultimately rejuvenating it and allowing it to rebuild. In our fast-paced, eager-to-always-be-productive society, the PNS state of rest and rejuvenation is of paramount of importance for physical and mental health. But depending on your current stress levels, you could be in the agitated SNS state for part of every day or longer. We can use movement to disrupt the time we spend in "fight, flight, or freeze." Practicing the pairing of certain movements with breath builds a type of muscle memory in the brain that can create a state of relaxation. Over time, this state of relaxation can be induced in your daily life as the muscle memory develops. A simple deep breath is commonly employed by most yoga practitioners in times of stress. Add in some light movement, you can hit a "reset button" within yourself. Then, you are able to shift your perspective from the stress-laden response to a new perspective that is resilient, even in the face of the same situation. Using breathing this way helps countless people through difficult times in their lives. Employees who work under weekly deadlines will use breathing and back-bending at their desks to refresh. For people going through family issues such as loss or other extreme changes, a breathing exercise with a forward bend helps with letting go of the past and accepting the new present.

By varying our movements and incorporating breathing in all spinal movements, we build a robust nervous system capable of adapting to difficult life situations.

Yoga Poses as Balanced Movement

Yoga is most widely recognized as increasing strength and flexibility. Poses call on different muscle groups, including ones you might not ordinarily use. Weight-bearing poses especially build muscle capacity. Poses also activate joints to move in ways that most people don't encounter in day-to-day activities, gradually increasing or maintaining range of motion. Done with clarity of intention and the individual's needs and limits in mind, this activity reduces the risk of injury. Balance is a key benefit of yoga poses. The classic tree pose is one example, as is raising an arm, a leg, or both, from an "all-fours" position on hands and knees. Coordination and body awareness improve as you learn to explore the balance of effort and surrender that each pose requires.

You might expect us to guide you through a few yoga poses at this point in the book. However, we're going to refrain. Since we don't know your individual body or movement story, we can't prescribe which specific poses would be beneficial. Instead, we suggest that if you are new to yoga, look for a beginner's class with a well-trained instructor at your local studio, gym, library, or online. Find a class suitable to your fitness level and experience the benefits for yourself.

Making Room to Let Movement In

We've been speaking mostly about making our bodies resilient by increasing movement in our daily life. One way we build emotional resilience is by examining our current habits and schedules and identifying what is and is not serving our health. By letting go of those things that do not serve us, we can create more room and energy to integrate habits that support our wellness, and yes—exercise and movement are essential things we need in our lives for whole-person health.

EXERCISE Strengths and Challenges for Increasing Movement

In this exercise, you will take time to establish your current set point: Where are you regarding establishing and/or maintaining a regular exercise routine? Be gentle with yourself as you go through this exercise and refrain from judging yourself. We all have both strengths and challenges and taking time for objective observation creates an opportunity to adjust where desired. Take a few minutes to consider the following questions.

- What does your current exercise/movement routine look like?
- Do you have a regular practice in place that uses one or more of the different forms of movement?
- Have you found it challenging to create and maintain a regular routine?
- Do you face particular challenges, including illness or injury?
- Is your job and/or daily routine active or more sedentary?
- If it's sedentary, are there little things that you do throughout your day to incorporate more movement, such as taking the stairs or getting up from your desk to stretch from time to time?
- Do the people in your life support and encourage healthy exercise and movement (including colleagues, friends, neighbors, family, etc.)? Are there environmental strengths and/or challenges? For example, does your work permit exercise or does where you live or any health conditions assist or detract from exercise?

Open your journal to a fresh page and draw a line down the center. At the top of one column, write "Strengths" and over the other, write "Challenges."

Under each column, write a list of strengths and challenges you identified from the questions.

Over the next few days, observe your routine and environment, considering where you can create opportunity to adapt or overcome some of the challenges you identified. Go into this with open and creative curiosity, understanding that some challenges may not change but others can. Small shifts and adjustments can make a significant difference over time. Use your strengths as a foundation to build from. Jot down ideas as you think of them.

In the next section, you will have an opportunity to take this information and create a daily routine.

Putting Your Potential into Action with Daily Routines

Yoga philosophy includes the concept of effort, discipline, or motivation as one of ten key guidelines to follow for putting our potential into action. However, this version of discipline relates more to action and activity than to forcing new behavior to become part of your life. There is effort required to gain some momentum, which is why a clear motivation is needed. Embracing discipline with a self-care mindset means that our relationship with discipline is cyclical. We have to look at discipline in the context of the rest of our lives; it's not a one-size-fits-all kind of approach. Rather, to be truly disciplined with an activity, it's important that it aligns with our preferences, needs, intentions, strengths, limitations, and energy. As you learned in the previous section, letting go of habits that drain your vitality will open up the space for you to reconnect with these aspects of yourself and invite joy and pleasure into the act of moving your body.

EXERCISE SMART Goals for Creating a Daily Routine

Throughout this chapter you have taken time to listen and establish your baseline, you have identified your strengths and challenges, and you have practiced reframing your mindset around exercise from one of punishment, if that applied to you, to that of self-care. Now, it is time to use what you have learned to incorporate this knowledge into your daily routine by establishing your goals.

Creating new or adapting behaviors to make positive change is often initially challenging as you develop new habits. Setting clear goals supports your success. SMART is an acronym: Specific, Measurable, Attainable, Relevant, and Timely. Throughout this book are several goal-setting exercises that follow the SMART goal-setting format.

- **Specific:** Be clear about what you want to achieve, when, and how. Consider limitations and relevant conditions. Identify why you want to achieve this goal.
- **Measurable:** What will it look like when you achieve your goal? Break the overall goal down into measurable parts that show concrete evidence of success.
- **Attainable:** Consider how to accomplish your goal and what resources are needed. This may include mindset shift, new skills, and life adjustments.
- **Relevant:** Is it worthwhile to you? Does it match your needs and desires?
- **Timely:** Set a realistic timeline for when you want to reach your goal, including a timeframe for short-term steps to take.

Take out your journal. Feel free to reflect on the previous exercises to support this process as you consider your goals for incorporating more movement into your daily routine.

- Where would you like to adjust your current exercise routine or add in new practices?
- What would you like to achieve through these changes? What are your goals?
- What is your motivation to make these changes? Improved health? Better sleep? Less stress? Increased stamina? Decreased pain? Recognize as many factors as are relevant to you and your life situation and make a note of them.
- What action steps can you take to make these changes? List all that come to mind.
- What evidence will show you that you have made progress?

- Are there any limitations that you need to compensate for in order to achieve your goal?

Using the SMART format, write out your goals in your journal. Identify the specific goal(s) that you wish to achieve and how. If you have more than one, prioritize. Determine how you will measure your success, both short term and overall. Establish what you need to attain your goal, including internal and external resources. Write out why this is relevant and important to you; get clear on your motivations. Lastly, establish a reasonable timeline for reaching your goal or goals. Be thorough but also have fun with this. You will find it easier to achieve success when you approach your goal with a positive mindset.

Chapter Summary

In this chapter, you learned how movement increases your physical health as well as your physical, mental, and emotional resilience. You examined your mindset in relation to external and internal motivation, as well as to the words "exercise" and "movement," exploring how that relationship may hinder or support your daily movement practice. As you learned to approach movement from a perspective of self-care rather than punishment, you created SMART goals for incorporating movement into your daily routine. We support you in following through on the goals you set for yourself here. It's a wonderful first step in practicing self-care for your body health.

In the next chapter, we continue with the yoga path of health and focus on the lifestyle category of nourishment.

four

NOURISHING YOUR WHOLE SELF

This chapter explores what it means to nourish your whole self. The Comprehensive Yoga therapy paradigm for nutrition includes more than just the physical foods we eat. Nutrition for the whole person considers everything we take in through our senses. From the images we feed our eyes to the sounds and words that enter our ears to the environments in which we spend time, we are continuously absorbing energy from the world around us. Once we are aware of this, we can become more discerning about the interactions that support our physical, mental, and emotional health.

From the Yoga philosophy term *koshas*, we learn that human beings are made of five sheaths or layers: body, energy, mind, intellect, and spirit. Each layer receives its own energy as we take in the outer world on many levels. We ingest carbohydrates, proteins, and liquids on the physical level, air via breath on the energetic level, sensory input and emotions on the level of the mind, ideas on the intellectual level, and inspiring spiritual principles on the level of the spirit. Each of us is unique, making you the expert of your own nutrition. Unlike many one-size-fits-all food or fad diet plans, Comprehensive

Yoga therapy empowers you to be the owner of your experiences, including your nutrition. Becoming familiar with the nutritional options that best nourish each of your layers is a key to cultivating whole health.

In this chapter, we will more fully explain the koshas and explore how we can use this philosophy as a framework for determining what is healthy nutrition for each of our layers, as well as how to bring balance to our whole being. The exercises and yoga practices will guide you to reflect on your relationship with nutrition and the factors that influence your current diet (that is, all the foods you eat). We will discuss yoga and the digestive system and Comprehensive Yoga therapy principles (not rules!) for wholesome, healthy nutrition. You will also create personal rituals before and after eating so that your whole self—all five layers—receives energizing nourishment.

Being Your Own Expert

In Western culture, especially in the media of the United States, we find an entire health industry revolving around weight loss. People wish to be slim for a variety of reasons such as personal image, social pressures, better energy, or longevity. Each of these goals may or may not lead to health.

Numerous dietary approaches, each claiming to be the best diet for healthy living, have created confusion around what, when, and how much to eat. Some approaches advocate for a certain food group while others claim the same food group to be unhealthy. Some diets encourage cooking (certain) whole foods while others require you to buy their premade, prepackaged foods. So much more could be said here about the do's and don'ts set forth by the diet industry and other dietary approaches but suffice it to say that the common denominator among them all is a set of rules that are assumed to be good for everyone. Yet, how can this be true if each human being is unique with different needs, preferences, histories, and health goals?

Rules are limiting and prevent us from discovering for ourselves what nutrition works best for our health and overall lifestyle. While some diet plans and approaches may offer valid points, Comprehensive Yoga therapy recommends that each of us learn and experiment to find out what provides us optimum energy and nutrition. In the case of a person with an acute disease condition, Comprehensive Yoga therapy recommends a consultation with a registered dietician or nutritionist to assist in this process.

Ultimately, we are the experts of our own bodies and lives. By learning to pay attention to our body's messages, not only do we empower ourselves to be the expert of our nutritional needs, we take ownership of our lives in a very purposeful way, integrating habits that work best for us and support our overall health. As we will discuss later in this chapter, yoga principles—which are different from rules—provide a foundation upon which we can stand as the expert of our own nutrition and health. Part of feeling confident in our ability to trust our internal cues is gaining an awareness of the external factors that contribute to mixed messages about nutrition. These factors, such as scientific research, the food industry, government, and the media, are multifaceted and complex. A basic understanding of the role these mechanisms play in messaging about food can go a long way in questioning and even debunking the rules they put forth.

The Role of Scientific Research

Research plays a useful role in nutritional health. It gives facts on the nutritional values of various foods and can offer input about the role of those foods in preventing disease and managing disease symptoms. Still, there is a limit to the utility of research, because scholarly scientific studies are not designed to tell *you* specifically as a unique individual what you should eat, how to be healthy, lose weight, or prevent or cure a disease. Instead, what researchers do is set out to examine a specific, well-defined scientific question. They may look at how a food affects the behavior of children with *attention-deficit/hyperactivity disorder*, for example, or if a popular diet has adverse effects on measures related to heart disease. A research study is carefully designed. The investigators may take measurements of a group, guide them through a change in diet, and then take measurements again to see if the intervention made a difference. Or they might compare two or three different groups, keeping everything about the groups as similar as possible except for the food or diet under investigation. From there, they draw conclusions based on the evidence they find.

In the rigorous rules of science, the conclusions only apply to the type of people and the specific food or diet being researched. If the study examined weight loss in heart disease patients over sixty years of age, for example, the results would only apply to heart disease patients over sixty. If you are forty-five and healthy, the results aren't intended to apply to you. And even for heart patients over sixty, the results are not a guarantee. Every individual is different. You would have to try the diet for yourself to see if it is appropriate and beneficial (with your doctor's approval).

Scientific studies also serve as guideposts to other scientists. When a study is successful, with intriguing results, other researchers will follow up to further the scientific knowledge. They might repeat the study to make sure the results can be replicated and were not an accident. Or they will vary the research conditions in some way to gain a little more understanding. Different researchers will study different related questions. Then, over time, the various studies are aggregated, and an overall picture emerges. But again, the results only apply to the situations that are studied.

Why Mixed Messages Exist

We know how science and scientific study provide us with evidence of possible advantages and drawbacks regarding certain dietary options for different groups of people. Unfortunately, the way in which the media communicates that scientific research often muddies the messages. In some cases, commercial interests and even the government become involved in confusing the information as well. One example of this is the low-fat craze that dominated American culture in the 1980s and 1990s. The low-fat idea began in the 1940s with a scientific finding that people who had cardiovascular disease often had a high intake of saturated fats and cholesterol. In 1961, the American Heart Association recommended that people who had heart attacks or had a family history of them reduce their intake of animal fat. The thought was that this change *might* lower the risk of heart disease, though their report cautioned, "…there is as yet no final proof that heart attacks or strokes will be prevented…"[6]

The idea that eating a very low-fat diet was healthy for everyone and not just heart patients began to spread. Twenty to thirty years after the initial report, seemingly everyone from physicians to the federal government to popular health writers unquestionably advocated for a very low-fat diet.

---

6. Ann F. La Berge, "How the Ideology of Low Fat Conquered America," *Journal of the History of Medicine and Allied Sciences*, Volume 63, Issue 2, April 1, 2008: 139–177. https://doi.org/10.1093/jhmas/jrn001.

The food industry responded to the trend by creating processed foods that were low in fat but high in sugar and other artificial flavors and additives. As a result, many people across the United States who followed the low-fat diet fad compromised their health by eating low-fat foods that lacked nutrition and were packed with unhealthy ingredients. Society's idea of the low-fat fad's benefits far outran the integrity of the science.

Now, a few decades later, researchers have learned a lot more about how fats work in the body. Their conclusions have led most health professionals to argue for a more moderate, nuanced approach to eating that includes a balanced amount of healthy fats.

Conducting Your Own Research

In general, Eastern medicine pays more attention to digestive health than we do in the West, regarding it as the crux of health. Learning to notice foods not just when they are on our tongues, but as they travel the whole way through our bodies can help us become aware of how we respond to foods. Paying attention in this way is how we gather data as we conduct our own personalized research. You can apply the following set of questions to any food you eat throughout the day, and we encourage you to keep a food journal of what you find, specifically examining how your food choices influence your physical, mental, and emotional health. You can refer to this writing afterward and learn from it.

EXERCISE Know the Effects of Food on Your System

To kick off your personal research study, we invite you to pick a food that you recently ate and answer the following questions. There are no right or wrong answers, so no need to censor your honest responses.

- Where did you eat this food?
- Did you take your time or were you rushed?
- Were you sitting or standing?
- What else were you doing while eating?
- How do you feel thirty minutes after eating (or drinking) the food?
- How do you feel two hours later?

- How do you feel the next morning?
- Do your insides feel at ease or uncomfortable when you eat this food?
- Do you feel energized or sluggish after eating this food?
- Do you feel mentally clear or cloudy after eating this food?
- Do you have an emotional connection with the food or notice any shifts in emotions after eating this food?
- What is your self-talk like about this food?
- How often are you eliminating? (For information about healthy elimination, refer to the Bristol Stool Chart online.)
- Is your elimination frequent and easy or infrequent, uncomfortable, or painful?
- Any other observations?

Keeping a food journal for three days to a solid month or longer will go a long way in revealing which foods offer you the greatest physical, mental, and emotional health benefits. (As with diets, some people are helped by a food diary more than others!) It will also help you identify habits around eating that might be worth changing or ending to better support your nutrition and overall health.

Understanding Food Relationships

Our personal relationships with food started before we were born. Culture, community, and economics shaped our parents' and grandparents' interactions with food, and some of their various attitudes and experiences were passed on to us. When we were babies and drank milk for the first time, a relationship combining sustenance and nurturing began, based on the most fundamental of needs.

Although we make our own food choices as adults, these deep familial roots may continue to influence our habits. Reflecting on your own food history can illuminate where new choices and habits are needed to nourish your total health. The following exercises guide you to examine how your childhood experiences influence your diet currently. If you like, write down your recollections or represent them through drawing. See if you can untangle the ways that your personal food history informs the food choices you make now.

EXERCISE What's My Food History?

Take some time to reflect on your past experiences with food. It may be helpful to write out your thoughts and reflections to help you see a clearer picture of how these experiences have shaped your current relationship with food. Consider the following:

- What were mealtimes like at home as you were growing up? What memories stand out in your mind?
- Where did you eat your meals most of the time? Whom did you share your meals with?
- What emotional associations do you have with your meals?
- What were you doing during your meals aside from eating?
- What messages did you receive from the people in your home environment about food and nutrition? From the media? From schools, spiritual communities, friends or other community members?
- What other influences affected your relationship with food?

As you consider these influences, write about your current relationship with food and how these past experiences affect you now. What beliefs do you hold about nutrition? How have your eating patterns been affected? Your food preferences? What else stands out to you?

As this exercise suggests, understanding your food relationships starts with reflecting on your past and continues with studying your behavior in the present and enacting change to meet your health intentions.

EXERCISE Recording Ideas for Change

Perhaps some ideas about changes you would like to make in your nutrition are beginning to surface. Writing them down will make them real and help you gain clarity on the direction you want to head in terms of your nutritional health. Based on what you have learned about yourself thus far in this chapter, make a list of ideas of changes and/or new habits you would like to enact related to nutrition. This also includes mental and emotional aspects of food and eating. This list will come in handy for later exercises in the chapter.

Nourishment with the Koshas

The yoga philosophy known as the koshas is a helpful framework for deter-mining how to enact healthful change to nourish your whole being. You are probably familiar with the idea of body-mind-spirit. Yoga elaborates this con-cept a little more, viewing the human being on five layers (*koshas*) from the body to the spirit/higher self. In addition to body, mind, and spirit, these five layers include life energy/breath (*prana*) and distinguish the lower mind from the discerning intellect. In order, the five layers are 1. body, 2. life energy/breath, 3. mind (feelings and lower thoughts), 4. intellect (wisdom and dis-cernment), and 5. spirit/higher self. Each of these layers exists within the next, like a collapsed telescope, moving from the obvious to the subtle. The layer of the body holds within it the life energy or breath. In yoga tradition, we are taught that breath contains life energy, the subtle animating force (*prana*). Within the breath is the mind. In this case, the phrase "the mind" refers to whatever is taken in through the senses, including feelings and how the personality interprets that information. The intellect is quieter and can be likened to the wise, witnessing self. It is the part of us that is able to discern between the ego's reactions and the reality of the higher self. The most sub-tle of these layers is the ineffable spirit—that still, abiding bliss of the higher self that lives within us all.

The outermost layer is made up of matter, or the physical body. The phys-ical body changes significantly over time as we age. We come to realize that we are more than just a body. Within the physical layer and of a slightly more subtle nature is the breath or life energy. The body affects the breath and the breath can affect the body. By developing conscious breathing practices, we influence this subtle relationship; this is the fundamental reason breathing is such a powerful component of yoga practice. When we breathe deeply into the diaphragm, the body relaxes and releases stress, yet when breathing is rapid and shallow, the body and mind become tense.

Within the life energy layer and even more subtle in nature are our sen-sory perceptions and emotional responses to external situations, which is the layer of the mind. When we are frightened, we gasp for breath or stop breathing altogether and the body becomes rigid or quakes. When we cry heavily, breath comes in short spurts and the body quivers. When we are con-tent, the breath is deep and slow and the body is relaxed. These states of mind have profound effects on breathing, in turn affecting the physical body. Even more subtle than the mind is the intellect. This is the discerning self, not mere intellectual prowess. The layer of intellect is the voice of wisdom that says, "I'm feeling anxious now, but this too shall pass." When we are connected to wisdom through the intellect, the breath is more likely to be peaceful regardless of external circumstances. Finally, the most subtle of all the layers is spirit/higher self, the bliss layer. This is the state of universal consciousness through which we are connected to all beings.

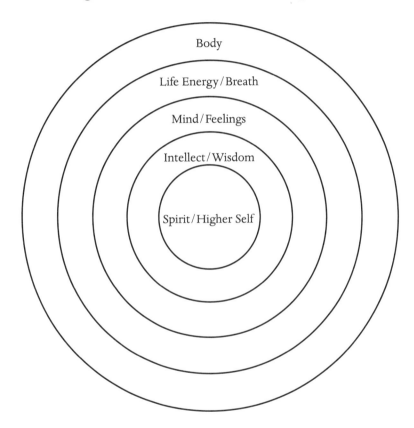

Figure 1: Koshas/layers

Nutrition and the Koshas

Throughout the day, we feed ourselves on many levels, and the food we eat has a relationship with all levels of our being. Our physical, energetic, emotional, mental, and spiritual states all influence our food choices. On the flipside, the food we ingest affects the health and sense of balance of all five koshas. Let's take a tour through the koshas and learn some possible ways to nourish each one.

Nutrition for the Physical Layer

In the last chapter, we talked about levels of energy called the *gunas*; they can also be applied to the classification of foods. Modern dietary programs would use this framework to group specific foods into categories usually to make one food group seem "better" than another, but that's not what we're doing. Instead, we are applying these concepts in relation to how food affects *you*, the person who ingests it, as an individual. Therefore, your chart will be as unique as you are. The effects of foods fall into one of three categories: pure (sattva), energetic (rajas), or dull (tamas) and can be characterized as:

Pure (Sattvic) foods:

- Digest easily
- Are high in nutrition
- Calm the mind
- Are bulky or heavy

Energetic (Rajasic) foods:

- Have strong tastes
- Stimulate the senses
- Are high in protein

Dull (Tamasic) foods:

- Lack nutrition
- Create a sluggish or depressed feeling
- Are heavily processed or overcooked

It is important to maintain a relaxed attitude toward nutrition. As you make different food choices, notice the effect those choices have on your energy levels as well as your mind. Whenever you are feeling particularly good or bad at any given time during the day, ask yourself, "What have I eaten?" and begin to correlate your food choices with your state of mind. Notice how making pure or sattvic choices begets balanced energy and healthier choices in turn. Likewise, observe any connections when your energy wavers. Develop an awareness of how foods would fill out your personal food chart, and let your newfound awareness inform your dietary choices. The food journal you began earlier in this chapter will be a helpful resource for tracking your energy.

Discovering proper nutritional habits is an individual process, which is why Comprehensive Yoga therapy avoids giving directions with specific diets or foods and instead offers more generalized advice: avoid processed foods, limit your consumption of refined sugar (including cane sugar, fructose, etc.), moderate or avoid caffeine, alcohol, white flour, and soft drinks. While complete avoidance may be impossible, it is not recommended to consume these foods daily. These "dull" (tamasic) foods disturb the digestive system and mental state and weaken the possibility for optimal health and well-being.

Ancient yogis understood that good digestion is a key to radiant health and is influenced by thoughts and emotions. The digestive system is a very sensitive mirror of the mind. Digestion is governed by the limbic area of the brain, largely beyond our conscious control. Emotions and mental processes act directly on the limbic area; via the nervous system, these processes affect the stomach and digestive organs. Thus the digestive system is solely under the influence of the autonomic nervous system. The parasympathetic nervous system (the mode of the autonomic nervous system that is dominant in a relaxed state) turns on digestive juices, speeds up peristalsis (the constriction and relaxation of intestinal muscles that move contents farther down the digestive tract), and opens the sphincters. Conversely, the sympathetic nervous system, usually in the form of a stress response, inhibits digestion.

Yoga poses are another way to nourish the physical body. When you press an area of the skin, it first turns pale, as the blood is pushed away, and then red as it rushes back. This is how yoga poses work on tissues; like a hand slowly and gently squeezing a sponge to remove all the stale, waste-bearing fluids, and then stretching the tissue to allow new life-giving nutrients and energy to circulate into the cells (see the nutrient cycle below). Yoga poses also massage the vital organs and stimulate the digestive muscles to increase their peristalsis.

A major benefit of doing yoga poses is that the entire digestive system is stimulated. As covered in chapter 3 on movement, work with a yoga instructor to learn how to move the body in all directions to stimulate the digestive system.

Nutrition for the Energy Layer

Proper breathing is one of the most overlooked aspects of health. Breathing is the only bodily system that we can control consciously. Rapid breathing stresses the body, whereas rhythmic, deep breathing balances the entire system. Some main benefits of deep breathing are increased blood circulation, increased carbon dioxide expulsion, relaxation, emotional stability, oxygen absorption, and increased energy. Physically, deep breathing boosts immune function by increasing oxygen metabolism, stimulating lymph propulsion and generation, and by improving the nervous system's interface with the immune system.

The ancient yogis observed that a person who is balanced on the physical, mental, and spiritual levels exhibits a strong life force or vitality. They named the life force *prana*. So *pranayama* refers to the mastery or control of the life force through the practices of breathing exercises and healthy living. Pranayama as a practice was developed based on observations made by these same yogis during deep meditation. They noticed that when they were in deep contemplation, their normal breathing pattern slowed down. They also discovered that the reverse was also true: by controlling the breath, the mind could be brought to a state of deep concentration. By learning to pay attention to your breath, you can become more aware in everyday moments, thus being more conscious in changing patterned behaviors and thoughts. Physical issues and even cognitive and emotional issues heal more quickly with the help of adequate breath.

Breathing corresponds to thoughts and emotions. If you are someone who is plagued by the stress of a mind that never stops thinking, you stand to be greatly helped by breathing exercises. The breath becomes the anchor that steadies the mind. Likewise, your emotions can be balanced by deep breathing. Both upsetting thoughts and intense emotions alter normal breathing patterns. By balancing and deepening the breath during times of emotional distress, you can find some relief.

Yoga Breathing Exercises for Digestive Health

Following are breathing exercises that aim to stimulate and increase the body's vitality by directing it to specific areas for special purposes, including healing. Breathing deeply during poses sends more oxygen to the cells and removes carbon dioxide, which has a powerful effect on the nutrient cycle. Here are a few breathing practices that you can use to nourish your energy layer.

- **Abdominal Breathing:** Stimulates peristalsis and relaxes the abdomen, essentially giving the practitioner an abdominal massage. Can be performed standing, sitting, or laying down. Slowly inhale, expanding your belly out like a balloon. Exhale, relax the belly back toward the spine. Repeat ten times.

- **Three-Part Breathing:** Building up the lowest area of the lungs is an important step to complex yoga breathing. Find an instructor who can help you move the intercostal muscles laterally at the rib cage area. Next, fill the upper lungs or the clavicle area, completing a deep breath. Remember that the exhalation aspect of breathing is the most important step. Removing the air from the lungs is the first step in proper deep breathing.

- **Breath of Fire:** Stimulates sluggish digestion. Inhale naturally and then exhale through the nose, as if you are trying to dry out water from your nostril. Let the inhale come passively as you forcefully exhale from the abdominal region. Repeat in rounds of ten.

Nutrition for the Mind Layer

The mind layer concerns the five senses and our reactions to stimuli, that includes emotions. The food for this layer can be divided into both intake and assimilation. We can learn to "feed" our senses with positive, uplifting experiences. We can also learn to reduce emotional dissonance by perceiving less sensory input. The modern world of technology can overwhelm our senses, which is akin to overeating for the mind. By filtering images that we receive and monitoring the input that we take in, we can reduce the burden placed on the mind and free up vital energy.

A second important area to consider is how we interpret the outside world. Much of the time, our daily reactions to commonplace things such as traffic or our neighbor's dog barking are based on our internal belief system, which usually classifies the world into "things we like" and "things we dislike." If you are a dog lover, you might feel a fondness for the barking from across the yard, while another person could feel annoyance. Knowing that you can alter your perception of the outer world can also be a way of minimizing upsetting responses you have to stimuli so they can become neutral or even positive.

Energy in all forms feeds the sheath of the mind. The five senses receive a voluminous amount of information each day. Your skin, tongue, nose, eyes, and ears are subject to a constant onslaught of data. Your mind filters these sensations and determines how to pay attention to relevant data. The information you receive is a type of food for the senses. When you are in situations where beauty surrounds you, the stimulus lifts the spirit. For some, a walk through a natural wooded area filled with nature's raw power soothes the senses. On the other hand, depending on your personality and disposition, a walk through a polluted, busy, and over-populated area can bring an abundant amount of stress into your system. Your mind must actively filter the unwanted sensory input. In small doses, this kind of environmental chaos is manageable, but we need to monitor what we take in on a daily basis to ensure that we as individuals are not over stimulating our minds and creating unnecessary stress or overload.

When we show outward kindness and other uplifting feelings for others, our digestive system among other systems in the body is benefiting. This development of a positive mood is felt throughout your body via the nervous system. It creates a sense of ease. Thus, being kind to another is also being kind to the systems of your body! While there may be some scientific studies discussing the effect of emotions on the nervous system, some phenomenon are proved by empirical study or simply common sense. When you are in a positive state, a happy state, there is a relaxed feeling throughout your nervous system. We don't need science to prove that positivity equals belly laughter, deeper breathing, and improved relationships. Considering that we know how prolonged stress has negative effects on the body, the absence of stress means a healthier system. Within modern life's intensity, it is good to be intentionally positive!

Ways to Nourish Your Mind Layer

- **Intake of Positive Emotions:** Rarely do we consider whether mundane activities are building up a positive reservoir of energy. List the types of activities that are uplifting to your emotions, such as keeping in touch with friends, playing with kids, enjoying the sunrise and sunset. If you have trouble with your list, start with simple things, e.g., a good meal or the kindness of your friends/family. Receive simple blessings from things like the sunset, appreciation of simple things like your meals, the fact that you have a place to sleep. For those of us who are blessed with plenty, it can be easy to overlook these simple gifts!

- **Gazing:** For the eyes, practice gazing. Attempt to look at a pleasant object such as a tree in the distance, the flame of the candle, or the moon. Relax the neck muscles and find a comfortable posture. Then, relax the muscles around the eyes until you gaze at the object with no emotion attached to the seeing. Let the image come to you and learn to remain at peace internally by developing an internal locus of attention.

- **Listening:** For the ears, practice listening to one sound only when many sounds are present. Choose one bird chirping, one instrument from a piece of music, or another pleasant sound. In time you will learn to filter all sounds except the sound of your choice. This skill can be translated into everyday situations by focusing your mind and allowing all other sounds to wash over you unattended.

Nutrition for the Wisdom Layer

The fourth kosha is the wisdom layer and refers to the essence of the mind found in the wisdom of the intellect. In order to care for the intellect in similar fashion to the mind, we can reduce sensory input. One of the ironies of the intellect is that it does more with less. A clear intellect is unencumbered by emotions, likes and dislikes, and other desires. To see deeply into your own intellect, it helps to be in a calm surrounding. A meditation practice declutters the intellect by supplying it with times of zero stimulation, allowing self-realization to develop.

Do you read books or other texts that help you discover the wisdom of the ages? By studying wisdom texts or philosophies that help you get at "the truth" of life, you help your intellect to navigate you through the vicissitudes of life. Relying on these timeless truths, the intellect hones the art of perception. In doing so, it can help to guide the mind as it copes with the emotional reactions we all experience. Due to past trauma, misinformed views of reality, and self-centered desires, the intellect can be hampered. The ultimate problem for the human mind lies in confusion between the spiritual and the material. Changes continually occur in the material aspects of life, and as soon as we forget this fact, suffering occurs. As the intellect processes sensory information, it shows us the change. When we cannot accept this change, we have emotional reactions that can be mild, medium, or strong.

For example, when you visit your old school, you will likely be struck by how you felt as a young student. The feelings may be good but they may have teenage angst in the mix. Some people may get caught up in the angst, feeling it as strongly as they did all those years ago. However, the mature intellect will rely on the wisdom that while old memories may resurface, they belong to the past. By knowing this play of the psyche, it is easy to remember that you are now a well-adjusted adult and maintain your emotional stability.

As you become more aware of how your perceptions are always trying to dictate your experiences, you get more chances to rely on wisdom and practice the skill of discernment. When you work to enlighten the wisdom layer with both meditation and spiritual study, you raise your intellect's ability to relate to life with wisdom. Via this wisdom, the layers of the mind and body are balanced and energized.

Nourishing Your Wisdom Layer

- **Read Inspirational Texts:** For one week, choose an inspirational book or scripture to read each day. Notice how the ideas permeate your intellect, reminding you to greet life with higher energies such as gratitude and kindness. With a clearer intellect, the mind's emotions are stabilized due to clear thinking. You may especially notice these effects if you do not already practice spiritual reading.

- **Meditation:** Practice meditation each evening to clear the mind by reviewing the events of the day in a neutral light, without judging yourself or others. Reflect on these events to find peace and sleep soundly thereafter. In the morning, take a few moments of quiet to plan your day and use prayer or visualization to guide your actions. By setting the stage for a clear mind, you save energy and make choices that strengthen health of the mind and body.

Now from this positive, enlightened intellect, we prepare ourselves to develop the next kosha, the bliss sheath, where complete fulfillment awaits us in every moment.

Nutrition for the Bliss Layer

The process of understanding the first four koshas ultimately brings us to the final kosha, the innermost sheath: the bliss body. This kosha is fed by activities that bring a sense of ease and contentment. When you are able to let go of all negative thoughts such as worry, fear, and doubt, a feeling of inspiration ensues. Endeavor to find a few truly inspiring activities. These should be personally meaningful to you; they do not have to measure up to some kind of spiritual "standard." It is the quality of the feeling and connection, not the outer experience, which dictates its connecting ability. This type of experience is the most potent means to achieving nourishment of mind and body.

Modern culture continually directs our attention to external events and objects in order to obtain happiness. The quest after earning excess money or power assumes that happiness lies in the material. The truth is that complete happiness resides within.

Remember that the koshas are all interrelated. When you feel inspired about life, the intellectual sheath finds the motivation to continue purification of the mind with meditation and/or other similar activities. As the intellect remains peaceful, the mind sheath is guided in emotional stability and moderate usage of the senses. A healthy mind leads to proper breath and vital energy. The breath invigorates the outermost sheath of the body. Finally, we have learned that our food choices reflect the state of the deeper sheaths.

Nourishing Your Bliss Layer

- Reflect on experiences in your life and continue to receive the gifts and lessons from those experiences. A profound moment that was either wonderful or difficult may be the source of spiritual development.
- Create something from your heart and without judgment: a poem, story, drawing, painting, or a dance.
- Spend time in nature appreciating the awesome beauty of life.
- Enjoy the company of animals or young children.
- Sit in the presence of teachers who inspire you.
- Go to a retreat to deepen your personal spiritual practice or seek connection with other likeminded individuals.
- Join your personal religious group or other community for worship, singing, chanting, and prayer.

Rituals for Before and After Eating
That Nourish Your Whole Being

Deep-seated rituals around food carry the weight of spiritual beliefs. To see this, think about times when you have been a guest at a meal. Notice how important the rituals are that surround food in this circumstance, how respectful you are as a guest of the food choices and manners of the host.

When you bring the habit of awareness to the table, you will develop an inner sense of what truly nourishes you. The habits suggested here target each of the layers and bring them into balance with one another. You might use these as suggestions and create your own rituals that feel nourishing and uplifting to you.

Before Eating
- Come to the table relaxed and with awareness
- Practice deep breathing to help become more relaxed
- Keep the breath slow and rhythmical while eating
- Take a moment of silence for appreciation and gratitude for the food and where it came from

During a Meal

- Remain aware of your body, breath, and mind

- Try to sit in easy pose or if you are in a chair, try not to cross your legs to let energy flow freely into the abdomen

- Remain fully aware of the process of chewing and swallowing. Each taste, temperature, and texture should be fully experienced—savor each bite slowly

- Don't watch TV or engage in lengthy, high-energy, or emotional conversations. Charged interactions may interfere with your digestive process and cause you to make less healthy food choices. (For example, mindlessly snacking while watching an engaging movie.)

- Chew your food ten to forty times before swallowing it, allowing the digestive juices in your mouth to fully interact with each bite as you enjoy its flavor.

- Experience the meal with full awareness: the pleasure of eating, the comfort of having plenty (but not too much), the energizing lightness that comes when the stomach isn't overly full

- Let go of fear—of weight gain or loss, eating too much, or being perfect or imperfect—by affirming your positive intention and your feelings of appreciation for your food

- Return to your breath and feelings of gratitude throughout the meal

After Eating:

- Remain aware that the food has passed down into your stomach and the digestive process is underway

- Sense the effects that the meal is having on your overall energy and perception of well-being

EXERCISE Meditations for Digestion

Each of the following may be practiced on its own or together to unite the mind and body in healthy digestion.

- Sit in hero pose or easy pose and try to become aware of your digestive tract. Visualize the digestive tract in your abdomen and become fully aware of all of its movements and sensations. Use your knowledge of anatomy to visualize ideal digestion in progress in your body. Look for images to help you if you've forgotten.

- Focus on the natural rhythm of your breath in the abdomen. The more relaxed and aware you are, the better your digestion will be.

- Visualize the sun with its center at your navel, radiating power throughout the whole of your body. Feel its warmth digesting the food and sending prana and nutrients to different parts of your body.

EXERCISE Your Nourishment Plan for Your Five Layers

To close this chapter, you will create your self-nourishment plan following the steps we outlined in chapter 2.

Listen

Now that you have learned about the koshas and various methods to nourish them, take some time to reflect on what you are currently doing on each level. What is working well for you? What isn't? Where would you like to see changes?

Learn

In your journal, create a page for each layer of the koshas. Go back and review the recommendations in this chapter. Starting small, pick one or two methods of nourishment that you would like to start applying, then write them down on the corresponding pages of your journal. Next, brainstorm about some other practices that you can use to nourish each layer. Be creative and have fun.

Love

Over the next several weeks, create opportunities to start using the practices you chose from this book or ones that you created. If needed, create reminders for yourself to help you as you begin working with these new tools. As you actively use each practice, remain mindful, open and curious. Notice how you are feeling as you use each one. What shifts do you sense in your body? Emotions? Thoughts? Energy? Which ones bring the most benefit? Are you noticing any internal resistance? Do you need to adjust the practices you are using? Continue adding practices that speak to you, exploring to learn what tools and practices most nourish each of your five koshas.

Live

Once you have explored several practices and tools, choose those that are most nourishing and supportive to you and build them into your routine. Create regular opportunities throughout each day to consciously nourish each layer of your koshas. Use reminders as needed to help you fully integrate these practices into your life.

By feeding yourself on all layers, you will notice your overall energy and sense of well-being improving. Health arises through the care of the whole person.

Chapter Summary

This chapter continued with the yoga path of health, focusing on nourishment. You explored a variety of exercises that nourish not just the physical body, but every layer of your being; the five koshas:

- Body: Nourishing your body through nutrition and food
- Energy: Learning to control your breath to nourish your energy
- Mind: Nurturing your senses with the conscious input of uplifting experiences, and the reduction of sensory input
- Intellect: Mastering your senses to manage your mental and emotional interpretations and reactions to sensory input
- Spirit: Connecting with the wisdom of your higher self to better discern between the reality of your higher self and the misperceptions of the material world

Through this exploration, you've had the opportunity to uncover habits, thoughts, and beliefs that hinder your well-being, as well as those that support it. As you apply these principles and practices to your daily routine, you provide nourishment for your whole being.

Next, we explore the lifestyle category of rest and relaxation.

five

HONORING REST
AND SLEEP

Like food, rest and sleep are nutrition for our whole self. Creating a lifestyle that honors rest and sleep is essential for physical, mental, and emotional health. Without enough rest, the physical systems of our body are affected, as is our mental clarity and ability to balance emotional responses.

Interestingly (but not surprisingly) sleep is not highly valued in our modern culture and society. There are no magazines at the grocery store checkout dedicated to sleep. We don't see celebrities promoting designer pajamas. No one is publicly praised for how skilled they are at sleeping. Rather, our society rewards productivity, action, accomplishment, efficiency, and success. Rest and sleep have somehow come to represent the opposite of those values. Still, if our society undervalues sleep, our bodies most certainly do not. A lack of sleep affects our mood, performance, and overall health. We add that lack of sleep even affects our relationships and finances, too. And when our attitude toward rest and sleep is one of resistance, we can form habits that negatively affect our health, such as working late to be productive, for example. Understanding your personal barriers to sleep—be they physical, mental, and/or emotional—is one of this chapter's goals. So before we begin the dialogue, let's examine your rest and sleep personal baseline.

EXERCISE Your Rest and Sleep Baseline

In this exercise, you are invited to look at your current patterns, habits, and beliefs regarding rest and sleep. Take out your journal to record your thoughts and insights as you consider these questions. Remember that this process is designed to help open your awareness and establish where you are so that you can see if there are areas you would like to change. Approach this with an open, curious mind; refrain from judgment.

Rest

- How do you define rest?
- How often do you allow time to rest each day?
- Do you feel you have time available to rest and relax?
- When you do have breaks or rest periods, how do you use that time?
- What do you feel when you have time to rest? Are you able to relax fully? Or do you experience some difficulty or resistance?
- What thoughts or beliefs do you have about taking time for yourself to rest?
- What activities do you engage in that help you fully relax?

Sleep

- How many hours do you sleep on average?
- How easily do you fall asleep?
- Do you sleep through the night or wake up occasionally or frequently?
- If you do wake up, how long does it take to get back to sleep?
- How do you feel when you wake up?
- Do you have a steady sleep schedule or varied?
- What is your bedtime routine and how does it support or hinder your sleep?

Next, review your responses to these questions. What are your strengths? What is working for you? Do you see areas that you would like to improve upon? Write it out in your journal to reflect on as you continue through the chapter. These insights will support you later as you create your sleep plan.

Sleep and Your Health

Let's start by looking at the many things that happen in your body while you sleep and why they matter so much for health—and there's no doubt that they do. Next, we'll examine why so many people have trouble with sleep. If you are one of them, you're in good company for sure! More than 35 percent of Americans are not getting the recommended amount of sleep on a regular basis, according to the CDC.[7] Forty-five percent of Americans say that poor or insufficient sleep affected their daily activities at least once in the previous seven days, reports the National Sleep Foundation.[8] And in a 2016 survey published by Consumer Reports, 68 percent of respondents struggled with sleep at least once a week.[9] We'll offer recommendations from science and considerations from Comprehensive Yoga therapy for integrating new habits and practices that support rest and sleep in your life and for your health.

In 2015, after reviewing an accumulation of scientific research, the American Academy of Sleep Medicine (AASM) and the Sleep Research Society (SRS) reported these eye-opening findings: Research shows that frequently sleeping fewer than seven hours per night is associated with impaired immune function, increased pain, impaired performance (such as at work), and greater risk of accidents. Getting inadequate sleep over time can lead to serious health conditions including weight gain and obesity, diabetes, depression, and even heart disease and stroke. Read on for information and self-reflective exercises to help you improve your sleep habits and thus your overall health.

---

7. "1 in 3 Adults Don't Get Enough Sleep," Center for Disease Control and Prevention (2016). https://www.cdc.gov/media/releases/2016/p0215-enough-sleep.html.

8. "Lack of Sleep is Affecting Americans, Finds the National Sleep Foundation," National Sleep Foundation (2014). https://sleepfoundation.org/media-center/press-release/lack-sleep -affecting-americans-finds-the-national-sleep-foundation.

9. "Why Americans Can't Sleep," Consumer Reports (2016). https://www.consumerreports .org/sleep/why-americans-cant-sleep.

The Power of Deep Sleep

Sleep puts our brains and bodies into an active recovery mode. To understand this better, let's do a quick biology review of a few body systems, starting with the endocrine system. This system consists primarily of glands—the pituitary, pineal, thyroid, thymus, and others—as well as a region of the forebrain called the hypothalamus; plus the pancreas and the sex organs, ovaries and testes. These glands, brain area, and organs all work together in a complex cascade effect, creating an intricate web of messaging that enables the body to (for example) regulate its temperature, feel hunger and thirst (and then stop feeling them after we eat and drink), and regulate sleep/wake cycles. The endocrine system is also responsible for metabolism, sex drive, muscle repair, and in children, growth and the onset of puberty. A complex and vital system, for sure!

The endocrine system does its maintenance and repair work during deep sleep. The amounts of hormones the system holds in "reserve" are checked, like gas levels in a car; and levels are replaced if necessary so the body is ready to function again the next day. Deep sleep is also when other systems do their repair work. It is when your endocrine system tells your immune system to replenish its supply of white blood cells, the substance that enables you to fight off infections and other micro-invaders, and your immune system responds. That's why you need to sleep more when you are sick; you need the time to generate additional reinforcements. Similarly, when the endocrine system signals the musculoskeletal system to repair itself (or grow, in children), both the endocrine "work order" and the physical muscle repair and growth happen during sleep. So you can see why sleep—and deep sleep in particular—are essential for health. If our bodies aren't asleep for a long enough time to generate the right amount of a hormone, the systems don't get a chance to work properly and health problems can result.

It's important to note that sleep is not the only factor in maintaining a healthy endocrine system. Genetics, behavior, and other factors also come into play, factors which can lead to endocrine diseases such as diabetes. However, science is increasingly learning that sleep is an important aspect of health.

As researchers are better able to study brain activity during sleep thanks to technological advances including functional magnetic resonance imaging (fMRI,) we learn more and more about the different ways sleep affects us. We all know that a lack of sleep can make one irritable, for example. Now we can begin to see that process work inside the brain. Though it isn't yet clear why, too little sleep compromises the brain's ability to adequately regulate and express emotions. It's exciting to think that in time, these finding may help doctors be better able to treat mood and anxiety disorders, including major depression and post-traumatic stress disorder (PTSD).[10]

Waves and Cycles: Stages of Sleep

Deep sleep is only one of several phases of sleep that occur each night. Scientists learned a great deal about the stages of sleep and wakefulness in the 1950s and 1960s by measuring brain activity using electrocardiogram machines (EEG), to record levels of brain activity through sensors affixed to patients' scalps.

There are three levels of waves: high beta, beta, and low beta, indicating varying levels of intensity. A normally active and awake brain exhibits beta waves. A student taking a tough exam, two friends engaged in lively conversation, a patient waiting in a doctor's office would each show the corresponding level of beta waves. The next level, alpha waves, are the indications of a person who is awake but at rest. Rest, like sleep, is a vital but undervalued experience. And also like sleep, our brains at rest may not be "idle" but very active. Some researchers theorize the existence of a Default Mode Network, a regular, baseline state of activity that the brain reverts to when it is not involved in goal-oriented tasks. In this more relaxed mode, they attest, you can reflect on your own and others' emotional states, make moral judgments, or muse on things that have happened to you (that is, memories) and things that might happen to you in the future. There is also a common belief that rest times allow for creativity, though this idea is not scientifically demonstrated.[11]

For most people (but not all), rest is a necessary stage before sleep. Once sleep begins, it happens in cycles, and each cycle contains several stages that happen in a predictable sequence. Each stage serves a different purpose. On

---

10. Andrea N. Goldstein and Matthew P. Walker, "The Role of Sleep in Emotional Brain Function," *Annual Review of Clinical Psychology* 2014; 10: 679–708.

11. Randy L. Buckner, Jessica R. Andrews-Hanna, Daniel L. Schacter, "The Brain's Default Network: Anatomy, Function, and Relevance to Disease," *Annals of the New York Academy of Sciences 1124*, (2008): 1–38. PMID: 18400922.

average, it takes a healthy adult 90 to 120 minutes to complete a cycle. The sequence of stages stays steady throughout the night, but the percentage of time in each stage changes. We all pass through numerous cycles each night depending on how long we sleep.

Stage 1: This is light sleep. Your eyes are closed, muscles are relaxed, and your body transitions from wakefulness to deeper sleep. This stage usually lasts on average for 15 to 20 minutes in healthy sleepers, that is, those who aren't experiencing insomnia or other sleep issues.

Stage 2: This stage is regarded as the true beginning of sleep. Now the senses are completely disengaged from their surroundings. Body temperature and blood pressure lower, moving toward deeper sleep. EEG activity at this stage shows a slow pattern, which is expected during sleep, but marked by sudden bursts of activity known as sleep spindles and K complexes. Researchers believe these kinds of brain activities serve two purposes: one, to help you stay asleep in the face of noises or other activity that might otherwise wake you. The other relates to learning, including both the cognitive learning of new facts, concepts, and so on, up to the mastery of motor skills. Specifically, researchers believe that during this stage of sleep, your brain sorts through the information and experiences you took in during the day, prunes out what is unnecessary, and transfers the rest to long-term memory, where you will be able to access it. As one would expect, school-age children experience long periods of stage 2 sleep.

Stages 3 and 4: These two are associated with non-rapid eye movement (NREM) sleep. These two stages are often grouped together because they are the periods of slow wave sleep (SWS).[12] This is the most restorative stage of sleep, consisting of delta waves, or slow brain waves. It's often difficult to awake someone in this stage of the sleep cycle. Sleepwalking, sleep talking, and night terrors occur during the deepest stage of sleep. EEG readings at this stage show long, slow brainwaves indicating deep,

---

12. Mark Aramli, "5 Stages of Sleep: Your Sleep Cycle Explained," February 8, 2017. https://bedjet.com/blogs/sleep-blog/5-stages-of-sleep.

restorative sleep. This is the time when the maintenance and repair discussed earlier happens.

After a period of roughly 30 to 40 minutes in deep sleep (again, on average), the process reverses itself. Sleep moves back to stage 2, where it is a bit lighter and the brain waves begin to look more active. But instead of moving back to stage 1, this is when the brain enters dream sleep.

REM Sleep: Called REM (Rapid Eye Movement) sleep, this dreaming stage looks completely unlike the rest of sleep. During stages 2, 3, and 4, circulation, respiration, blood pressure, and body temperature all decrease. But as you enter REM sleep, all these measures begin to rise. Brain activity increases so much it is sometimes more active even than during the waking state. Your eyes dart back and forth, quite possibly to survey the dream images created in the brain. The only thing that doesn't increase activity is your muscles. Instead, they become temporarily paralyzed. Surprisingly, this paralysis has a practical advantage—for normal sleepers, it keeps them from trying to "act" out or move as they would in their dreams … a good thing! During an eight-hour sleep period, you will have four or five rounds of REM sleep, with the last round lasting an hour or more.

Have you ever wondered why you dream? Many researchers believe dreams have a role in creating memories. One theory, the Contemporary Theory of Dreaming, holds that dreams are the result of connections being made and unmade within the brain, guided by the emotions of the dreamer. From a scientific perspective, however, why we dream remains a mystery.[13]

Valuing Rest in Your Life

As discussed earlier, modern life rewards us for achievement. And a somewhat ironic example that shows this perfectly is in the healthcare field. Obviously, suffering patients need care, but this often means that doctors, nurses, and other healthcare professionals are required to forgo their own sleep to pull long hours and double-shifts, routinely working well over eight hours

---

13. Ernest Hartmann, "Why Do We Dream?" *Scientific American*, July 10, 2006. https://www
.scientificamerican.com/article/why-do-we-dream/.

per day. These long work hours have become a badge of honor and are simply expected in the field. The same is also true in business, law, IT—so much of our work life demands time that ends up robbing us of sleep. A second area where rest may be needed relates to any activity overdone in life. While some are dedicated to their careers (or to saving their job), there are others who love to exercise seven days a week. Some artists have gone days without eating while in the midst of an intense creative surge, only to crash for days afterward.

EXERCISE What Are Your Beliefs About Rest?

Take out your journal to record your thoughts and insights as you consider these questions.

- What does rest mean to you? Do you rest?

- How does your profession view rest?

- How did your parents demonstrate rest? Was a family member called lazy for resting, or was rest connected to laziness?

- Do you view rest as something relegated to one day a week, or do you have a regular routine? Be inclusive when considering what a rest routine might entail—some might consider dog walking as a form of mental rest.

- Do you ever take a rest or "fast" from screens?

- How do you wish to reframe your view of rest?

A Relaxation Exercise for Rest:
Contraction and Release Practice

The Contraction and Release practice helps to consciously relax different muscle groups by first contracting them and then releasing and relaxing the muscles, activating the parasympathetic nervous system. Let's begin.

Sit or lie in a comfortable position and begin taking a few slow, gentle breaths. Notice how your body feels, recognizing where you feel tension and where you feel open and relaxed.

With each muscle group, take a long, deep breath in through the nose as you contract the muscles. Hold the breath and the contraction to the count of four, and then slowly and gently release the breath and the contraction simultaneously to the count of four. Go through each group one at a time, working your way down your body:

1. Close your eyes tightly

2. Clench your jaw

3. Raise your shoulders up toward your ears

4. Pull your shoulder blades together in your back

5. Clench your fists, bending your arms and bringing your fists up tight against your shoulder or upper chest.

6. Contract your abdomen, pulling the muscles inward toward your spine

7. Clench your hips and thigh muscles, bringing your upper legs together

8. Flex your feet, bringing your toes toward your head

9. Press your feet away from your body, pointing the toes

For the next 5 to 10 minutes, remain where you are and breathe gently and slowly, allowing your body to relax more deeply.

Developing Healthy Sleep Hygiene Rituals

Even before you get into bed, you can create rituals to prepare yourself for rest and sleep. Below is a list of recommended "sleep hygiene" habits based on the National Institutes of Health's *Your Guide to Healthy Sleep.*[14] These suggestions are a good place to start when considering small but significant steps you can take to improve your sleep.

- **Stick to a sleep schedule.** Experts advise against sleeping in on weekends. The body loves habits, and it responds better to a consistent bedtime and rising time. Additionally, sleep time cannot be "banked" for later, a phenomenon known as "sleep debt." That is, being short one

---

14. "Your Guide to Healthy Sleep." US Department of Health and Human Services, National Institutes of Health, National Heart, Lung, and Blood Institute, Publication no. 11-5271. Originally printed November 2005, revised August 2011. https://www.nhlbi.nih.gov/files/docs/public/sleep/healthy_sleep.pdf.

or two hours of sleep every weeknight cannot be "made up" by sleep-ing extra hours over the weekend.[15]

- **Get enough sunlight.** Morning sunlight especially helps set a good pat-tern for sleep later on.

- **Exercise, but not too late in the day.** Daily exercise helps sleep, but exercise too close to bedtime can make sleep more difficult. Notice the degree of exercise's effect on your sleep: too much exhausts and depletes the body, too little creates a restless feeling.

- **Don't nap after 3 pm.** Naps can help make up for lost sleep, but naps that are too late in the day or too long make it harder to fall asleep the next night.

- **Avoid caffeine in the afternoon or evening,** and avoid nicotine. Both are stimulants that interfere with sleep.

- **Look at your medications.** Some commonly prescribed medicines and over-the-counter remedies interfere with sleep. Talk to a doctor or pharmacist about whether what you are taking could be causing sleep problems. Ask if it is permissible to take them earlier in the day.

- **Avoid large meals and beverages late at night.** A snack is okay, but eating a lot at night can cause indigestion that can keep you awake. Beverages too close to bedtime cause awakening to urinate.

- **Avoid alcoholic drinks before bed.** While they may help you relax, they keep you in the lighter stages of sleep, robbing you of deep sleep and dream sleep.

- **Relax before bed.** Leave time in your schedule for winding-down activities.

- **Create a good sleeping environment.** Limit light, especially from screens. Keep the room temperature cool. Your pillow and mattress should feel comfortable. Turn the clock away from you and keep your

---

15. Katherine Dudley, "Weekend catch-up sleep won't fix the effects of sleep deprivation on your waistline" Harvard Health Publishing: https://www.health.harvard.edu /blog/weekend-catch-up-sleep-wont-fix-the-effects-of-sleep-deprivation-on-your -waistline-2019092417861. Posted September 24, 2019.

phone on silent and out of reach so you don't stress about what time you're falling asleep.

- **Don't lie awake in bed.** If you can't fall asleep and are getting anxious about it, move to another location to read or listen to music, or engage in another relaxing activity.[16]
- **If you still can't sleep, consider seeing a doctor.** Doctors can diagnose sleep disorders and other medical causes of sleep difficulty.

Yoga Practices to Prepare for Rest and Sleep

There are various reasons why so many of us have trouble falling asleep. For example, sleeplessness can be a symptom of clinical anxiety or depression, and menopause frequently causes sleeplessness in women. But most of the time, the answer for why so many of us have trouble sleeping begins in our nervous systems. Your nervous system is your body's built-in alarm, guarding you from danger. It constantly asks the question, "Am I safe?" If the answer is no, it will release the hormones that prepare the body to run away or fight. If you lie in bed rehearsing the day's problems or anticipating the ones you expect tomorrow, you are basically telling your nervous system that no, you aren't safe. And your nervous system can only do is its job—keeping you awake, alert, and ready to act.

The key, then, is to switch the nervous system from the on-edge, fight-or-flight, sympathetic state, to its opposite—the rest-and-digest, parasympathetic state. By convincing the system that yes, you *are* safe and everything is okay, you are more likely to be able to relax and fall asleep. Yoga practices that downregulate the nervous system can be very helpful in preparing your body for rest and sleep. Conscious relaxation practices such as yoga nidra and meditation help train the nervous system to downregulate and prepare for sleep. Our nervous systems thrive on routines, so building solid yoga practices as part of your routines can be very beneficial.

Here we offer a few more ideas for downregulating yoga practices that you can incorporate into your sleep routine. We encourage you to take time to explore what works best for you. Record observations in your journal

---

16. This is the official recommendation. However, deep breathing, stretching, meditation, and other activities that directly relax the body can be done in bed.

about how these practices feel and what you notice physically, mentally, and emotionally as a result of doing them. Your journal can also be a place to record thoughts, worries, and other things on your mind that may interfere with calming your nervous system for sleep.

Gentle In-Bed Stretch

When the sympathetic nervous system is engaged, muscles tighten so the body is ready to move. Gently stretching before bed—or in it—helps the system to relax. Like the Contraction and Release practice on page 86, the intention of this exercise is to allow your body to relax and prepare for sleep. Drawing your attention to the breath and the muscles brings the added benefit of pulling it away from the mind. This gives you a chance to detach your mental focus from whatever is occupying it, allowing your thoughts to drift into the background.

Once in bed, laying on your back or side, inhale slowly and deeply as you extend your arms up toward the headboard or wall behind you. At the same time, stretch your heels or the balls of the feet toward the footboard or opposite wall. Stretch languidly in both directions, creating length in your entire body, then exhale and relax.

You can hold the stretch for several breaths, perhaps putting extra emphasis on extending your right arm and leg, and then your left. This will release the muscles along your sides. Once you release your stretch, it might feel good to wiggle around a little, or you could curl up; whatever feels the best to your body. Repeat the stretch if you like, perhaps widening your arms out to the sides this time.

Extended Exhale Breathing Practice

Many breathing exercises help with deep sleep, rest and relaxation. One easy exercise is to simply prolong and observe your exhalation.

Try this exercise lying on your stomach in a comfortable manner that suits you, or lie on your side if necessary. Breath in deeply, feeling your abdominal area press against the bed. Then, expand the rib cage area as you inhale further, ending in the upper chest.

As you begin to exhale, measure the breath to release as slowly as possible. Make a hissing sound if it helps you concentrate. The slow breath has a calming effect.

After a number of breaths, you can notice a deeper relaxation if you feel a gentle wave flowing up the spine as the contour of the breathing pattern moves the spine in a rhythmical manner.

Gratitude Practice

Practicing gratitude is a wonderful way to uplift your spirits and reduce stress levels. When you focus on those things that you are thankful for, your attention shifts away from things that worry you and towards things that are positive in your life.

You might want to get a separate notebook or journal and designate it as your "Gratitude Journal." Each night before bed, spend a few minutes acknowledging things that you are grateful for and list them in your journal. You can choose how many you want to list each day; ten is a common number. The key to being successful in this practice is to feel your appreciation for each thing that you list. Although there may be times when you are struggling and find it difficult to identify things you are grateful for, still make the time to make your list and do the best you can to connect with the sense of appreciation. You can start with very simple things such as:

- I have a roof over my head
- I have people who care for me
- Someone held the door for me at the store today
- I have a job that helps me pay my bills
- I have clothes on my body
- My colleague helped me with a project
- The sun is shining
- The rain is nourishing the plants
- I have a bed to sleep in
- I have food to nourish my body

It may help to focus on a specific thing or area of your life. For example, list five to ten things that you appreciate about your body, home, job, neighborhood, nature, or a specific sense.

- I am grateful for these five things about my body:
- I appreciate these five things that I see:
- I am grateful for these five things about my job:

Additional Gratitude Practices:

- Instead of a journal, create a gratitude box or jar; you can even decorate it if you're feeling crafty. Each day, write your list of things that you are grateful for on a piece of paper, fold it up and put it in your jar.
- Whenever someone does something kind, take a moment to fully feel and appreciate the gesture.
- When someone compliments you, accept it instead of deflecting it.
- Make a list of things that you appreciate about yourself, and maybe hang it up where you can see it.
- Write notes of appreciation to loved ones, friends, and colleagues. You can give them to the person or place them in your gratitude jar.
- Think back on challenging past experiences and identify how they benefitted you. For example, maybe they opened you to a new opportunity, helped you learn something valuable, taught you compassion, or introduced you to someone important.
- When you have a meal, take a moment to fully appreciate everything that made it possible for you to receive the meal and the benefits it will give you. Consider the farmers, delivery people, and grocers who created the food and brought it to where you could buy it; your job (or someone else's) that created the income to pay for it; and the person who prepared it, whether it was you or someone else. Pretty amazing to think about, isn't it?
- Look for opportunities to feel truly grateful for people and things in your everyday surroundings throughout each day.

EXERCISE Creating Your Own Ritual

You can nurture yourself and improve your sleep by developing a nightly sleep ritual. Set a specific time to go to bed each night and stick to it. Here are some other ideas of things to build into your ritual.

- Include your daily hygiene routine as part of your ritual. Build in mindfulness and gratitude practices as you do each step.

- Turn off all screens at least sixty minutes before bedtime.

- Dim the lights and lower the thermostat.

- Make a list of things that you need to do the following day and set it aside, so you don't have to think about them while you're falling asleep.

- Spend quality time talking with your loved ones.

- Take a warm bath or shower.

- Drink a warm caffeine-free beverage such as hot water with lemon and honey or warm milk.

- If you are worried about something or ruminating, write it out on a piece of paper or in your journal to clear your head.

- Meditate, pray, or practice mantras.

- Read a book or some poetry.

- Do some gentle stretching or yoga.

- Write in your gratitude journal.

Once you identify the steps in your personal sleep ritual, create a timeline and do your best to be consistent with it. Consistency will help train your brain to recognize that it is time to unwind and prepare for sleep as you go through your ritual.

Additional Comprehensive Yoga Therapy Considerations

Simple lifestyle changes can go a long way in helping with sleep and all areas of your life. In addition to integrating some (or all) of the sleep hygiene recommendations and other suggestions above, the considerations below can help you derive a greater awareness about your unique needs. They'll help you figure out what you need to put in place in your life to get the best possible night's sleep!

- **Pay attention to your sleep and rest** for a few days and really tune in to how you feel. How much sleep do you get if you don't set an alarm? How much sleep do you need to not feel sleepy during the day?

The seven hours quoted at the beginning of this chapter is the minimum amount of sleep recommended but remember there are individual differences. You might need less, you might need more. Many people need eight or even nine. And don't forget to leave extra time to relax enough for sleep to happen.

After waking in the morning, give your body a moment or two (or a few more) to equilibrate before getting out of bed. This gives your heart rate, breathing, temperature, and other body systems a chance to return to their daytime rates before you rush into your day.

• **Try a nap** if you do feel sleep deprived; it might help you feel rested and more alert. The key is to wake up within about twenty minutes (when you are still in light sleep), or at about ninety minutes (when you will have finished a complete sleep cycle). If you won't wake up on your own, set an alarm. Sleeping for a length of time longer than ninety minutes could wake you during deep or REM sleep and leave you feeling unpleasantly groggy and disoriented. Also, follow the suggestion about not napping after 3:00 pm (or another time appropriate to your daily schedule if it's unusual).

• **Learn Relaxation.** If naps don't work for you—and they don't for everyone—simply rest. Stop what you are doing for twenty minutes and engage in one of the exercises described earlier, or another activity that will relax you. Disengage from screens. Close your eyes if you like. Make the room quiet or listen to music or nature sounds. Resting allows your brain waves to slow down, giving your brain a break even if it's not getting the benefits of full sleep. (You'll also find more suggestions in chapter 11, on meditation.)

• **Monitor screen time.** Experts caution against screens before bed; take their advice seriously. Studies show clearly that screen time in the hours before bed interfere with falling asleep and is adversely associated with sleep outcomes.[17] The evidence shows that after looking at screens, nighttime body temperatures remain higher than normal and less of

---

17. Lauren Hale and Standford Guan, "Screen Time and Sleep Among School-aged Children and Adolescents: A Systematic Literature Review," *Sleep Medicine Reviews* 21: 50–58. June 2015.

the hormone melatonin is released.[18] Both of these changes interfere with falling asleep. Also, the precept from chapter 4 that what we feed our senses affects our health certainly applies to scrolling through social media or reading news articles on devices while in bed. Falling asleep this way could influence the quality of your sleep, the content of your dreams, even your mood when you wake up in the morning—a sort of negative-energy hangover.

- **Consider leaving your phone to charge outside of the bedroom.** Buy an old school alarm clock if you need it to help you wake on time.

EXERCISE Your Personalized Plan for Rest and Sleep

Take out your journal and refer back to your baseline exercise on rest and sleep. Here, you explored your mindset and established your strengths and challenges in these areas. Next, you are going to develop your personalized plan based on those insights and your exploration of the practices throughout this chapter. Using the SMART format learned in chapter 3, write your goals in your journal for rest and sleep. Consider the following:

- What habits and practices are currently working well for you?

- Where would you like to see improvement in your rest and/or sleep habits? Set specific intentions/goals about each of these.

- How will you benefit from these changes? More energy? Better mood? Less irritability? Clearer mind? Less anxiety? Be specific and list as many as you can think of.

- What is your motivation to make these changes in your routine? How will the benefits that you listed improve your life? Remember to refer back to your original intention from chapter 1.

- How will you recognize your progress?

- Identify practices, rituals, and routines that you will begin using to help you achieve your goal.

- What other resources are available to support you?

---

18. A. Green, M Cohen-Zion, A. Haim, Y. Dagan, "Evening Light Exposure to Computer Screens Disrupts Human Sleep, Biological Rhythms, and Attention Abilities," *Chronobiology International* 34(7): 855–865. May 2017.

• Are there any limitations that you need to overcome? What steps can you take to address them?

Once you have a clear plan in place, begin implementing your plan and building your chosen practices into your daily routine. Refer to your journal as needed to help you stay on track. Reach out for support if needed.

Chapter Summary

In this chapter, you learned the important health benefits of adequate sleep and the risks associated with insufficient sleep. Most people require seven to nine hours of deep sleep to maintain good health. You explored recommended practices and habits to employ that improve overall sleep hygiene, as well as Comprehensive Yoga therapy tools and practices that support relaxation and better sleep. In completion of this chapter, you developed your own personal sleep hygiene ritual and incorporated that into your personalized plan.

The next section on social health explores the lifestyle factors of work, relationships, environment, and finances.

part three
SOCIAL HEALTH

At our current point in human history, the Industrial era is barely 250 years old, and many places on earth still live an agrarian or outdoor, non-technological lifestyle—a way of life that is about 10,000 years old. In our recent history, pollution, disease, and global warming have developed. The number of social changes that have transpired in the past few hundred years alone are probably more than took place for the average human in the previous 10,000 years or even longer. We have managed to use factory mass production, increase population, and alter the temperature of the earth. The yogis have a saying: "Humanity can fly to the moon but doesn't yet understand their own mind."

This section on social health covers how these mammoth changes have made present day "advanced" people (that's us) true beginners in an exponentially changing world. And we haven't even discussed those handheld computers that have completely absorbed young and old people alike—the smartphone—or the artificial intelligence that burgeons on the horizon in greater and greater levels.

Chapter 6, "Transforming Work Stress," covers how to find harmony with work that oftentimes has little to do with the natural world. For many, day jobs are only a means to an end. This sort of disconnection leads to stress or unhappiness that leads to imbalance of health. The lessons here help you reclaim a conscious and even joyous participation in your work.

Personal relationships are another area to resolve, understand, and accept so that your emotional health can move in fulfilling directions. Chapter 7 relates the power of strong relationships to personal health.

In Chapter 8, involvement in and understanding of the need for the natural world is recommended. It's even proven with scientific evidence that shows how important nature is and offers recommendation for integrating nature into your life for physical, mental, emotional, and spiritual health. We explore how our bodies themselves are also nature, making all of us intimately connected to the earth and the air we breathe.

Lastly, the social health area that gives most modern humans the most stress of anything is old-fashioned coins, gold, cash—whatever you use to trade with others for goods and services. In a specialized world where people no longer grow their own food, money is used for everything. Chapter 9 will give you some valuable insights to find peace with currency and see how an enlightened attitude can bring you better health.

six

TRANSFORMING WORK STRESS

In the same way the yogic path of health offered guidelines for taking care of your physical body, the yogic path of work offers clear direction on how to transform daily work stress into a more rewarding relationship with the tasks of your personal and professional lives.

This chapter will guide you to examine how your relationship with work impacts your health. We'll start with research on work and stress and then offer ways we can move our bodies to relieve the physical stress of working, especially at a desk. Then we turn to the central concept of finding meaning in work and learn how to apply the precepts of karma yoga—acceptance, concentration, excellence, and nonattachment—to our twenty-first-century lives. Next we turn our attention inward, to the deep beliefs and blocks that materialize as stress and other states negatively impact our health. Finally, because work relationships often create much of the rewards and the stresses in our work lives, we will discuss a bit about the yogic perspective for healthy ways to relate to the people encountered at work.

Why Is It So Stressful?

Forces large and small combine to cause the tidal wave of work-related stress that we humans can experience. Changes in the economy and increased corporate financial concerns translate into long hours, heavy workloads, and demanding bosses. Fears about unemployment, business failure, reduced income, and loss of health insurance are widespread and very real. At home, chores and childcare require many hours of work even while their importance is dismissed or downplayed in society's general opinion. Responsibility for chores can cause significant friction between couples.

Unfortunately, job stress is a recognized source of health issues. These can be more minor disorders including pain in the neck or hands, eye strain, and difficulty sleep, ranging all the way up to serious issues of hypertension and heart attack. These conditions are very common all because of stress.

What if instead of relating to work through the lens of stress, all of us could embrace work as a path to health and well-being? Most of us are required to earn a living and all of us are required to do some work in our personal self-care and households. Wouldn't it be wonderful if you could learn to transform the stressful elements of work into more meaningful and even uplifting experiences? What great benefits could this bring to your physical, mental, emotional, and spiritual health? The rest of this chapter is dedicated to helping you transform work stress into opportunities to improve your health in all areas of your life.

Attitude also explains why the experience of work-related stress is highly individualized. A job that one person loves doing can be decidedly stressful for another. Often in a group of people, there are those who love certain household chores over others. Some find peace in folding laundry while other people's linen closets are disorganized. Some of us love to cook and make tremendous meals but know nothing about growing food, while the gardener may be happy eating her produce raw. In the case of tasks at work, there are few people who like paperwork over the actual human interaction aspect of their jobs, but there are days when being undisturbed doing paperwork is a better choice. Many healthcare professionals report that they enjoy working with patients. However, paperwork is considered annoying to the professional who has to document their work; they didn't sign up to do paperwork, they signed up to save lives—so the inner narrative goes. Hence, the stress around paperwork exists because of the lack of interest of the professional and not because paperwork is inherently stressful.

What if instead of relating to work through the lens of stress, all of us could embrace work as a path to health and well-being? Most of us are required to earn a living, and all of us are required to do some work in our personal self-care and households. Wouldn't it be wonderful if we could learn to transform the stressful elements of work into more meaningful and even uplifting experiences? What great benefits could this bring to your physical, mental, emotional, and spiritual health? The rest of this chapter is dedicated to helping you transform work stress into opportunities to improve your health in all areas of your life.

EXERCISE Your Work Baseline

In this exercise, you'll begin looking at your current thoughts, patterns, and beliefs related to work and how they affect your emotional state and your stress levels. Use your journal to record your insights as you consider the following questions. As a reminder, approach this exercise with an open, curious, and judgment-free attitude.

- As you think about your work, notice your inner dialogue. What thoughts come up? Do you notice that you have any repetitive patterns of thought about your work? Or do your thoughts about your work change based on specific situations you deal with?

- Notice how those thoughts impact your emotional state. What do you feel as you think about work? Is it a good, neutral, or unpleasant feeling? Perhaps a mix of feelings?

- Tune in to your body as you think about work. What changes do you notice, if any? Does your body feel at ease or tense?

- Identify aspects of your work that you find challenging—physically, mentally, or emotionally. (Keep in mind that challenges are not inherently negative. Sometimes challenges can be enjoyable, uplifting, or empowering.) How do these challenges affect the way you think or feel about your work?

- What do you value about your work? Consider the various aspects and identify those things that are enjoyable to you, that feel satisfying or perhaps even inspiring.
- Describe the purpose of your work. What is the broader vision?

Once you've finished, go back and read over your responses. What stands out to you about your relationship with your work? What do you notice about your mindset and thought patterns? Is it supporting your well-being or increasing stress? Use the awareness gained from this exercise to determine where you are currently so you can envision where you would like to go. What are your current strengths and assets? Where would you like to invite change? Write your insights in your journal and keep them forward in your mind as you continue through this chapter. They will help you formulate your personal goals for reducing workplace stress.

Easing the Physical Stress of Sitting All Day

Work for many of us means sitting too long in front of a computer screen, leading to a host of minor health problems such as body soreness, aches, and pains. Over time, living with chronic soreness and aches in your physical body increases emotional distress and decreases your quality of life. Referencing back to the koshas, or our five layers of being, tension in our muscles (physical layer) creates restriction in breathing (energy layer) leading to emotional angst (mind layer). Day in day out, our intellect thus becomes clouded, and we might start to make poor choices regarding self-care … or the lack thereof. For a common example, many people use unhealthy food as a reward, disregarding nourishment. In extreme cases, the strain or pain we experience physically prevents us from doing the activities that we enjoy (bliss layer). Our world becomes smaller as the physical discomfort and emotional distress increase. Attending to your body a little bit each day, even while at work, can help ease the physical and emotional stress of sitting all day.

The first step is equipment that supports your body properly. Do your best to use a chair that fits you. Your feet should be flat on the floor, with knees pointed forward and hips at an approximately 90-degree angle. A standing desk or adjustable desk is another great option, as well. Align your keyboard, monitor, and mouse so they are straight ahead of you with your elbows at a 90-degree angle and your eyes looking forward and a bit downward. The screen should be arm's length from your face. Make liberal use of devices such as bookstands to hold source material, along with wrist and elbow rests. From time to time while you're working, stop what you're doing and take a mental scan of your body. Is it in the position described above? Being mindful of your posture during the day may alleviate future problems. Research is catching up to the long-known truth that yoga poses are a great remedy for ailments caused by the strain of too much sitting. But you don't have to wait for a class. Following are two exercises to try. One study recruited a group of people to participate in a weekly yoga class and follow a yoga DVD at home for eight weeks. Another group received no intervention. At the end of the time period, the yoga group reported significantly lower scores for perceived stress and back pain, as well as sadness and hostility. Although these studies are of a small sample size, they do show promise for something that most of us find to be the case—that movement is an important aspect of health and that modern life sorely lacks proper physical use of the body.

EXERCISE Stretch Break!

It is likely that you are reading this book in a seated position, so first observe your posture. Most of us read and sit in a mild forward bend, sometimes leaning the neck forward. Take a moment and move your body in five directions so your spine awakens and reminds you to sit in a comfortably upright position:

- Lift your arms above your head to stretch in an upward direction.
- Twist from side to side while keeping the spine upright.
- Lean forward and release any tension in the neck and should area.
- Lean backwards with a nice breath to open the body.
- Lastly, move to the left and right for a side bending exercise.

Note that you can do these poses seated or standing, or even while taking a walking break.

EXERCISE Body Tension Scan

Throughout your workday, pause for a few moments and tune in to your body. Notice the cadence of your breath. Become aware of your posture. Tune in to different parts of your body and notice where you are carrying tension:

- Are your shoulders reaching up toward your ears or rounded forward?
- Teeth clenching or jaw feeling tight?
- Low back rounded?
- Head hunched forward?
- Tension around your eyes or in the forehead area?
- Clenching your fists or holding your equipment too tightly?

When you find areas of tension, stop for a moment. Exhale. Breathe slowly in and out. Stretch out the affected body parts. Straighten your spine. Pull your shoulders down toward the floor and roll them in small circles. Bring your shoulder blades together in the back to open your chest. Move your head gently forward and back, then side to side to stretch your neck muscles. Open your jaw wide and move it back and forth. Spread your fingers as wide as they can go. Roll your wrists gently. This might be a great time to get up and walk around for a few minutes.

Outside of work, make up for sedentary time by making sure you take plenty of opportunities to move. Consider taking a yoga class or following a video. Turn back to chapter 3 on movement and resiliency for more ideas about moving your body to counter the effects of too much sitting and other work-related tension.

Meaningful Work, Working with Meaning

All types of work have the potential to be meaningful, even spiritual, depending on the approach you bring to it. With the right attitude, you can find satisfaction and meaning and unite with your sense of spirit at work and in home tasks every day. By cultivating a spiritual attitude toward work, you'll be able to connect more deeply to your life, even the parts that seem to cause stress.

The path of karma yoga (the yoga of work), first mentioned in chapter 2, teaches us that all actions, even those as menial as washing dishes, are opportunities to connect with meaning and our personal purpose for doing that work. If we perform the work without the perspective of a higher purpose, we feel burdened and eventually resentful. The yoga philosophy of work brings us into awareness of our higher purpose for doing that task and invites us to complete any task with ease and peace of mind. The four-step yoga philosophy of work is:

1. Acceptance
2. Concentration
3. Excellence
4. Nonattachment to results

This approach offers a process for removing the burden of stress by keeping your internal purpose vital and top-of-mind while you work

Acceptance

The first precept of this method is to cultivate acceptance for the task at hand. Cultural norms and our (let's face it) typically self-centered approach to life create internal barriers to acceptance. We all have conversations going on in our own heads, referred to as the "inner voice." The next time you begin a task, whether at work or home, tune in to your inner voice. What is it saying? Is it functioning as a guide or a supporter, encouraging you along in your work? Or is it arguing and complaining?

Practicing acceptance starts with striving to make your internal voice work with you instead of against you. Start by trying to see the task itself as neutral. Say to yourself, "I am mowing the lawn." Period. Don't let that inner voice add negative judgments, like how your neighbor has a much better lawnmower than you do, or how someone else in your family should really do this job. Those things might be true, of course, but deal with them later. For now, your job is to do what you have to do with a calm, clear head.

It's important to note that acceptance does not mean passive tolerance. This is an unfortunate misconception. Accepting the fact of a situation does not mean you have to acquiesce to anything unfair, certainly not unethical or illegal. However, often when we deem something unacceptable, like a disliked task, a rude boss, or a disgruntled customer, we skip the acceptance step because we wish to deny that this is our reality. Yet we know that denial doesn't change the situation, it only saps us of energy and makes the situation more stressful than it has to be. When you practice acceptance instead, you feel accomplished and at peace. Too often a cryptic message can lead to a misunderstanding, or a tweet or an internet post may lead to snap judgments. The accepting step is meant to measure our reactions so that we have time to clearly assess a situation.

Acceptance also applies to work situations that are out of your control. You work for hours on a report and your boss changes her mind about how she wants it done; or you rearrange your schedule for a new client who cancels at the last minute. It's normal to react with frustration to these kinds of scenarios, but what is superior is to understand the roots of the emotional response within yourself. When these types of events come up, as they inevitably will, take a few deep breaths. Remind yourself that things like this happen. Accept the current situation as it is. Make the effort to understand your emotions so that the situation will teach you about your inner judgments, freeing you to be more open-minded, even peaceful.

Many people employ a strategy of positive thinking to accept things they don't like. Consider this scenario: You are on your way to a business meeting or taking your son to the doctor. You're late, and there is unexpected traffic. To accept the traffic, you try to be more positive. "Well, it gives me a chance to listen to my podcast." Or "I get to spend a little time with my son." Or "I am grateful that I have a car and the money to maintain it." All of these are better than futilely swearing, waving your arms, and honking your horn, but they don't lead to true acceptance. You have to keep expending energy on your positive thinking; when you stop, your negativity will likely return.

Practicing acceptance means adopting a neutral mindset toward reality, known in yoga philosophy as pure thinking. In this example, a neutral, accepting response would simply be: "Traffic exists." That's it, it's a fact, it has no inherent emotion. The emotion comes from the judgments and opinions about traffic we create in our own minds. Yes, there will be consequences. We may be late. But that, too, is just a statement of fact. Any negativity about it comes from our attitudes, not the actual traffic.

In case you're skeptically raising your eyebrows, let's start with a less loaded topic: Organic yogurt exists. You might like yogurt or not, but that preference comes from you. The yogurt is simply there. The same principle applies to traffic. One line of yoga thinking says that every situation is neutral; it is always our judgments, biases, and preferences that label them "good" or "bad." This can be a difficult concept to process. Of course we can all name things we deem unequivocally bad, like war or famine. That said, try to keep this possibility in mind, as it is a very useful concept for reducing stress at work.

In some cases, acceptance is the first step toward finding a resolution. Letting go of your biases clears your mind to envision a solution to problems or issues that are bothering you at work, whether that means an innovative change in procedure or advocating for fairness. Approaching colleagues and supervisors with a neutral attitude gives you the advantage of communicating your ideas calmly and rationally. Your manner will give you more credibility in the workplace and make it more likely that your objectives will be achieved.

Concentration

Concentration is the second precept of the path of karma yoga. In this context, concentration refers to focusing solely on the task before you. If we're mowing the lawn, we think only about mowing the lawn. We can use our senses, noting the difference in the grass height as we move along, smelling the freshly cut grass. We can bring in gratitude, feeling grateful for the growing grass, for our material resources, the beautiful day. Or if we're washing dishes, we might notice the feel of the dish soap and the water. We can contemplate the combination of material and human effort that went into creating the dishes and installing the sink, the technological wonder that allows for indoor plumbing.

Concentration sounds deceptively easy. We all know that our minds wander. We think about the other things we have to do, yesterday's work meeting, the morning's news. But imagine how much more aware of the world you would be—not to mention how much more grateful and content—if you could focus on just one thing at a time.

EXERCISE Concentrate on One Task

So why not try it out? For just thirty seconds, try to focus completely on one task. When (not if) you notice your mind wandering, acknowledge that fact and simply draw it back to your task. Make this a practice. Keep at it over a week or a month, perhaps adding a little more time each day to your concentration session. By clearing out distractions, concentration is a practice that has the potential to transform your outlook and decrease your stress, because you will feel pulled in fewer directions at once.

Concentration may seem like too quaint a concept for the twenty-first century. There's so much to get done, and technology allows us to accomplish more work in the same amount of time. Unfortunately though, studies show that this isn't true. Despite our devices, our old-fashioned human brains just don't have much ability to process more than one thing at a time. You might swear by multitasking, but research shows that when we switch our attention back and forth from one task to another, we become less efficient, not more. Our brains have to go through a cumbersome series of shifts that waste mental energy.[19]

Instead, experts recommend finding a quiet place to work, keeping your workplace clear, and only turning on one device at a time. Assign specific chunks of time for tasks that would otherwise encourage interruptions, such as checking email.

Paradoxically, our brains crave novelty and reward multitasking, which makes the habit extra hard to break. Consider setting an intention for yourself to replace the modern ethic of constantly chasing down mental stimulation with the traditional yoga notion of concentration on one task using the mind, senses, and spirit—the whole being. Start with small micro-goals to change your behavior, focusing on one very small change at a time. Reward yourself for each success.

Excellence

Excellence, the third precept of the path, means striving to do our jobs to the best of our abilities. This sounds familiar and straightforward; to a point, it is,

---

19. Earl Miller, "Here's Why You Shouldn't Multitask, According to an MIT Neuroscientist," *Fortune* magazine, December 7, 2016. http://fortune.com/2016/12/07/why-you-shouldnt -multitask.

but there's more. In yoga, excellence refers to doing your best at your tasks while balancing the overall picture. For example, if caring for your family is your job, excellence means doing that well while fitting in self-care. Remember that Comprehensive Yoga therapy means attending to your *whole* self. It sets priorities as self, family, work, and community, in that order. If you spend all your hours tidying your house, chauffeuring your kids, and volunteering at church but you don't have time to exercise, that isn't excellence. Maybe it would be better for you to join the Y and cut back a bit on volunteering. The same goes if you put in eighty hours a week at the office but neglect your family. Rather than overdoing one area of life to the cost of health and healthy relationships, excellence requires working on all tasks and responsibilities with balanced effort.

The reason for correcting these types of imbalance has to do with the meaning of work. To the yoga way of thinking, all work serves a greater purpose. Another aspect of excellence is to identify and pursue that meaning, whatever that means for you. The overall purpose may or may not be specifically what you get paid for or your job description. You might need to look at the bigger picture. Food shopping may be a drag, but it is a cog in the machine of keeping your family nourished and healthy. Or your purpose may lie in something tangential to your job, like bringing joy, friendship, or compassion to your coworkers' lives.

A parable from India makes the point well: Once upon a time, a kingdom faced a terrible drought; the farmers could not work their fields. To keep the farmers from being idle, the king put them to work building a new temple. Three farmers were crushing stones in the quarry to lay the temple foundation. A stranger passed them and asked, "What are you doing?" The first farmer scowled and answered, "The king commanded me to work like a slave, crushing stones in the hot sun." The second farmer said, "The king is paying us to crush stone. I have to do it because I can't make a living this year as a farmer." The stranger asked the third farmer, who smiled. "Can't you see, friend? I'm building a temple."

Like the parable demonstrates, the attitude we bring to our work is a choice. When we combine a neutral attitude with a commitment to internal excellence—a sincere endeavor to do our best—there is something inherently rewarding about giving a task our all.

It's necessary to point out that excellence is not the same as perfectionism. Excellence is an internal state of mind whereas perfectionism is an excessive focus on the outcome of a task. When you approach work with excellence, you feel the satisfaction of connecting to the experience of doing your best.

EXERCISE Excellence Check-in

As kids, we are taught to be honest, listen to our teachers, earn good grades, and try our best in all activities. As adults, we are to work hard, be team players, and achieve our work goals.

- List the standard view of doing a great job.
- What is excellence for you?
- What do others affirm in you?

Now think of this version of yogic excellence in terms of your state of mind.

- In the societal expectation that measures our value based on achievement, how does that feel to you? For example, is it pressure and effort, maybe sprinkled with some fear or drive? Another combination?

Now, examine applying your measure of excellence to an internal state of mind while simultaneously doing a solid job. Bring your intention into the work, notice how that feels. And, notice how you can still achieve great heights while remaining internally inspired.

Nonattachment to Results

Do your work with acceptance, concentration, and excellence; then, when you have finished the task, let it go completely. It's out of your hands. This is the essence of nonattachment, the fourth precept of the path of work, and the key to a stress-free work life. By practicing nonattachment to results, we can be at peace in every situation. Having the satisfaction of knowing we performed the task with excellence, we can be assured we did our absolute best, and that is truly all that matters.

The opposite approach—excessive focus on the result and how it will be received by others—creates stress in our bodies, thoughts, and emotional responses. It's very common in this situation for people to confuse their self-worth with the outcome of their work. When you hitch your sense of self-worth to the unpredictable ride of other's responses, it only makes sense that you would feel anxious, edgy, and stressed. Nervous systems shift into fight-or-flight mode. Health suffers in the short-term, and it's possible to develop more serious difficulties over time. Nonattachment allows us to keep our minds and bodies steady, strong, and secure.

The harder we work on something, the more passionate we are about it, just as the more we stand to gain from something, the more likely we are to ride the up-and-down waves of stressful anticipation. But no matter how hard you work, it may or may not pay off. The sale might or might not go through; the client might or might not accept your recommendations; the patient might or might not get better. Your children might or might not remember your instructions or take your advice. Nonattachment says to do what you are able and take pride in your efforts. Then, when you can do no more, it'll be better to view the results from a distance with a sense of healthy detachment.

We have been conditioned to expect rewards for jobs well done, some-thing that begins early in life with gold stars and grades in school. In this mindset, the work itself can become less important than the effects of the work. The yogic path of work reminds us that the greatest, most sustained rewards are internal. The only thing we have control over is our internal state and the degree of excellence we apply to our efforts. When we concentrate on what matters most and do our best, we can detach from the rest and free up so much energy for other, more nourishing activities.

To summarize, the yogic path of work begins with acceptance of any situation, considering how it fits into the larger reality. Full concentration is applied to the task. Through this focus, our best efforts arise. Excellence relates to the state of mind while working, as well as job performance. Lastly, we remain nonattached to the results of work. Nonattachment reminds us to enjoy the job for its own sake and not for the end results. Since we cannot control what happens with our work once it is out of our hands, we do not need to carry stress about the end results.

Putting the Path of Work into Practice

The following exercises will help you begin to apply acceptance, concentration, excellence, and nonattachment in your attitude toward work. Come back to them often as you continue to apply these philosophies in your life. Remember, decreasing work-related stress is essential to your physical, mental, and emotional health. Improving this area of your health will have wide-reaching ripple effects in other areas of your life.

Create a Mantra

As you work, focus on acceptance, concentration, and excellence. Afterward, remind yourself that you have done your best, and that's all anyone can do. Find words to articulate that thought in a way that resonates with you and repeat it whenever you find yourself getting tied up in results or outcomes. Many successful versions of this approach will acknowledge your limited control. Some people express it as giving the work over to God or the universe. Another version is, "What will be will be." You might write down your mantra and post it in places that are visible throughout your day.

Focus on Self-Development

Set an intention to be more empathetic or choose another virtue that is appropriate for you in your workplace, perhaps kindness, fairness, or courage. Especially for people new to their jobs, focusing on learning and skill-building works well. Then your identity becomes tied to pursuing a virtue or learning, instead of on the outcome of the work. Just remember to be compassionate to yourself in those efforts, as well.

Share the Responsibility

Remembering all the people and steps involved in the job you do allows you to see that, while you play a role, the success or failure of any venture rests widely on many shoulders. Even jobs that feel solitary are the result of a series of efforts. Educators who develop and deliver a lesson usually do so by themselves; but behind them are all of their own teachers who helped them learn their jobs; the staff, administrators, and ancillary workers who keep the school running; and the parents and students themselves, who ensure the educator has someone to teach. Extending out further are the people who created the books and other materials that served as resources for the lesson, and even the desks and chairs the students sit in. Regarded in this wide-angle scope, it is much easier to separate ourselves from the results of our labors.

Bringing Your Spirit to Work

What are some small random acts of kindness you can do at work? Can you do these kind acts with no need of recognition, simply doing it from your heart? How can you support others at your workplace? Can you see the bigger picture for your job and how your company makes a difference in the world? Even stay-at-home parents run important "companies"! Can you determine your value from within and speak kindly to yourself?

Internal Obstacles

Acceptance, concentration, excellence, and nonattachment lay out an aspirational blueprint for an ideal way of approaching work, one that allows us to be both outstanding workers and happy, healthy people. In practice, though, obstacles block the efforts we make toward achieving that goal. By learning to change your perspective, to direct your mind along different paths, you can be your own best hope for rising above. When we master our minds, we conquer everything about our work situations, leading to better work results and better, more healthful selves. Reaching these heights usually requires digging down into our subconscious minds, learning more about our reflexive thinking, and changing it to better suit our goals.

"Change" in this context refers to true, enduring change, not quick fixes that don't last. Equipping yourself to make those changes means diving under the surface a bit of your own psyche. At times what you discover will be benign, an unconscious expectation or thought that you didn't realize was influencing your behavior. At other times you might need to delve deeper, possibly uncovering difficult emotions. In these cases, we recommend working with a qualified psychotherapist to help you through.

As a first step, in the moment of anything you find stressful related to work, remember that relaxation exercises described throughout this book are always available to you. These techniques work best if you rehearse them at home when you are already relaxed; then you can call on them even in the middle of your workday. Use whatever is your favorite, such as breathing slow, deep breaths into your belly; or focusing on the feel of the breath as it comes in through your nose and goes down your throat. Try bringing a calming image to mind, perhaps the beach or a mountain. Or repeat something to yourself in your mind. It could be a mantra, a short prayer, a sound from nature, or calming music.

EXERCISE Hidden Influences

Each of us has past experiences, beliefs, and needs that influence our behavior and emotions. These often work below the surface, unconsciously guiding our actions and reactions to life experiences. Through developing awareness of these underlying influences, we are empowered to make conscious choices about how we respond to life, rather than remaining controlled by emotional reactivity to circumstances and the behaviors of others.

Oftentimes, when something occurs that is contrary to our underlying beliefs or reflective of a past experience, we become triggered and react in a manner that is disproportionate to the circumstances in front of us. We may become very upset, angry, anxious, or fixate on the situation. These physical and emotional reactions are indicators that there is an underlying influence driving us. Internal inquiry helps to identify the hidden influences that are causing the reaction.

In this exercise, you learn to build your internal awareness as a tool for tracking your physical and emotional reactions to external circumstances. As you become aware of your internal reactions, you then have the opportunity to go deeper and identify what is causing the reactions you are experiencing. Use your journal to record your experience and insights. Initially, you will begin by looking back on recent situations to help you learn the steps and build your awareness. As your internal awareness increases, you can begin using these steps in real time to override the reactivity and learn to instead respond to life situations from a place of deeper consciousness.

1. Recall a recent experience where you became irritated, angry, or upset with a person or situation. How did you respond? Tune in to your body.

   a. Notice the thoughts that arise as you think about the situation now.

   b. What were the thoughts as the situation occurred?

    c. Become aware of how your body feels currently.

        i. Do you feel tension anywhere?

        ii. Notice changes in heart rate or breathing?

        iii. Sensations in your abdomen or chest?

    d. What were you feeling when it happened?

    e. What emotions arise now?

2. Where does your reaction come from?

    a. Can you identify what is causing your reaction?

    b. Does it remind you of a past event?

    c. Is it challenging a belief?

    d. Are your needs not being met somehow?

    e. Do you feel you are being wronged in some way?

    f. What is the story that you are telling yourself about this situation? Take your time with this and get clear on the underlying influences of your reaction. Remain aware of your thoughts, emotions and physical sensations as you go through this inquiry. Notice judgments, resistance, or tension. Jot down any insights you gain.

3. Once you've identified what is influencing your reactions, take another look at the current situation from this new perspective.

    a. What can you reframe about how you interpret this situation?

    b. Use the practice of pure thinking that you learned previously to identify more neutral thoughts about the situation.

    c. Take note of what shifts in your body as you do this.

Plenty of situations arise at work that might trigger a deep-held belief, so how do you know which ones to analyze this way? The basic answer is, anything at work that causes you significant emotional discomfort is a likely spot to look. What causes your muscles to tense, your throat to close, or your stomach to churn? Is there something similar about these situations? Your answers are fertile grounds for self-discovery. As well, you might notice external cues. Something is probably triggering you if your reaction is more extreme than other people's.

Consider trying out this process of examining your beliefs. You could do it just in your own mind, by talking it out with a friend or writing it down in a journal. Think of a person or a situation that pushes your buttons. Start there and follow the steps listed above. If the emotions become too painful, consider talking it out with a trusted confidante or a therapist. Some of our expectations, such as that people should behave ethically, serve a useful purpose to help keep ourselves and others acting in socially acceptable ways. Sometimes we can uncover our hidden beliefs and unconscious biases and decide that the situation is still unacceptable if it crosses deeply held values. In that case, a two-pronged approach might be necessary; you can take whatever steps are in your power to change the situation while at the same time doing what you can to protect yourself from stress.

Unconscious Biases

Unconscious biases are one type of underlying belief that set up expectations of how people should act in a particular job. They can apply to everyone around us and to ourselves. We all have expectations that people in certain work roles or situations should behave in certain ways. Often our expectations have far more to do with our personal experiences and preferences, and less to do with what the job really requires. We know how we think things ought to be done and we think everyone should do them our way. But inevitably we will run up against people or situations at work who don't live up to our unconscious expectations. This is common among young people who land their first jobs and discover that in the "real world," things don't always operate as cleanly or ideally as they were taught in school. But it happens to all of us.

In these cases, we usually have two choices: We can allow the other person's style to disturb us and cause us stress, or we can change our own perspectives about what is acceptable. It bears repeating that this doesn't mean accepting unfair, unethical, or illegal behavior. It means adjusting our mindset to the wide variety of possibilities that exist for acceptable ways to work.

And what about your unconscious beliefs and biases about yourself at work? Are you holding yourself to impossible standards? What does it mean to you to be a good employee, or teacher, salesperson, or mother—any job title you hold? Does it mean being available 24/7? Never making a mistake? Fixing everyone's problems? Give yourself permission to apply the same understanding, empathy, and common sense to yourself that you apply to others when you are being your best self at work. In that way you will benefit your work, your relationships, and your own physical and emotional health.

EXERCISE Reframing Your Mindset

Let's look at how your mindset affects your stress. Take out your journal and look over your notes from the previous exercises in this chapter. Notice any trends related to how you think and feel about work. Do you have a positive mindset, or do you create more stress through negative thoughts? As the new work week approaches, do you automatically dread it, anticipating that it is going to be difficult? For example, is Monday always presumed to be a bad day even before it happens?

Self-Observation

Over the next week, observe your statements and thoughts about work and make note of how you feel. Do your thoughts feel heavy, overwhelming or stressful? Or do you feel light and relaxed as you speak or think about your work? When you hear others bemoaning their job, do you join in and agree with them? Make notes about your observations. At this point, you need not change anything. Just observe and notice your thought patterns.

Reframing

Open to a new page in your journal and draw a line down the center to create two columns. Based on your prior journal entries and observations, write a list of your thoughts and statements that promote stress in the first column. In the second column, write a more neutral or supportive statement for each.

Example: "Ugh! It's Monday! I hate Mondays."

Reframe: "Monday is just a day. It is neither good nor bad. I have the opportunity to create the kind of day I want to experience," or "It's the start of a new week. I'm setting my intention to make it a good one!"

Example: "There's Mr. Late to the Office again. He earns the same salary as me …"

Reframe: "Mr. Late has young kids and thus he is late due to helping them get to the school bus. I will now call him, Mr. School Bus Dad."

EXERCISE Your Personalized Plan for Work Stress Transformation

You've learned how work-related stress impacts your overall health and well-being and explored yoga practices and principles to counter stress and improve your health. Next, you are going to create your personalized action plan using SMART goals to apply these principles and practices to your work situation. Refer to your journal notes from this chapter as you create your plan.

- What specific changes would you like to make to improve your work experience? Set specific intentions/goals.
- What work habits and practices are already in place that work well for you?
- Where do you see opportunities to make changes to help reduce work-related stress?
- How will you benefit from making these changes? Less tension? Decreased stress? Greater satisfaction in your work? List anything you can think of.
- What is your motivation to make these changes and achieve your goals? What will you gain and how will your life improve?
- How will you identify that you are making progress?
- Identify specific practices and tools that best apply to your needs and create a plan to incorporate them into your routine.
- What other resources are available to support you? How will you access them?
- Are there any limitations that you need to overcome? What steps can you take to address them?

Once you have a clear plan in place, begin implementing your plan and building your chosen practices into your daily routine. Refer to your journal as needed to help you stay on track. Reach out for support if needed.

Chapter Summary

In this chapter, you explored multiple levels of stressors commonly associated with work. You practiced exercises to reduce stressors that derive from physical demands of your job, internal beliefs and attitudes, and interpersonal interactions. Additionally, you discovered how to apply the path of karma yoga to your work by practicing:

- Acceptance: holding a neutral mindset about work
- Concentration: maintaining sole focus on the task at hand
- Excellence: striving to do your best on each task
- Nonattachment: letting go of each task after completion and being unattached to outcomes

You learned to alter your belief patterns and expectations of situations to transform a charged situation into a neutral one. Thus, you stop stress at the inception point by altering your internal mindset. The exercises and practices in this chapter provide tools that empower you to transform your work experience from stress to bliss.

Like the journey at work, our preconceived notions of relationships can cause us repetitive issues with family, friends and even ourselves. In the next chapter, we focus on how to create health in our relationships.

seven
BUILDING STRONG RELATIONSHIPS

We are social creatures; we need one another to survive. Babies thrive with contact and touch from others. Kids develop through play with other children. Adults marry, form families, and preserve extended families, often enduring tensions to keep the relationships alive. The power of relationship runs to our core as it did from when we were all once tiny babies dependent on caregivers.

Think of how powerfully relationships affect you: How do you feel after a wonderful night seeing old friends? How do you feel when gathering with others in your preferred form of divine worship? Likewise, do you feel exhausted from a tense time at work or a spat with your friend? One upsetting interaction can negatively impact your day and cause your nervous system to spiral out of control until you feel exhausted by the afternoon.

Before we go into the various benefits of relationships and discuss some of yoga's interventions to your relationships, let's listen to your own story so that you can have a clear sense of your relationship dynamics. This exercise is extremely important to fill out; you might skip others, but putting your relationship cards in front of you might be the most powerful part of this entire chapter.

EXERCISE Your Relationship Baseline

List the five most important relationships you have in your life. But instead of using names, use groups. For example, list "child" or "children," "parent" or "cousin," and so forth.

- How do you benefit from these five relationships?
- What are your personal criteria to determine if you have healthy relationships?
- On a scale from 1 to 10 with 10 the highest, rate your relationships in terms of their health.
- In what areas are these relationships lacking or where is improvement needed?
- How does your family of origin's dynamics influence your view of relationships?
- Do you view your relationships from an emotional standpoint? Or do you view relationships from a spiritual, intellectual, or activity perspective, or a combination of any of these?

Relationships can cause people immense emotional problems when their expectations are not in accordance with reality. As relationships are a matter of the heart, the effects of any discord with the reality of a situation can turn lovers into vicious opponents in court or leave siblings not speaking to one another for years. Likewise, a relationship with healthy boundaries and awareness of boundaries can be a point of health, joy, and longevity. As we go through this deeply emotional territory, keep in mind that strong emotions may come up that would benefit from discussion with a therapist or counselor.

The Spiritual Significance of Relationships

Please understand that in this chapter we are glossing over the profound depths and nuances of relationships. On the surface, emotions may define relationships, but it is up to us to navigate the emotions lest they dominate everything, cloud our judgment, and overwhelm us. That said, emotions are just the surface area of a relationship in the way that lava is just the result of tectonic plates deep in the earth.

Once we start to accept the state of relationships and manage our emotions, we can start to see the underlying dynamics at play in our relationships. We can examine our deeper needs and our assumptions about how we think people should behave as they intersect with our biological need for loving dynamics with other human beings.

Problems occur when we seek the love and warm feelings from outside of ourselves. When I look to my friend or family member to feed my internal state of happiness, joy, or love, my life becomes completely out of control. This is the level of most relationships: someone is nice and I feel good; the same someone is upset and then I'm upset too.

In understanding what makes us tick in terms of our relational dynamics, we can finally uncover the truth and begin to understand the nature of those tectonic plates that exist deep within our heart. If I learn how to shift relationship dynamics so I see them as sparks that ignite recognition of my own internal stability that exist with or *without* another's mood, I am no longer dependent on outside factors that are uncontrollable. This is what is meant when spiritual teachers stress the importance of having an inner life or a higher self, or being grounded. Essentially, you define yourself based on the divine or nature, *not* on the emotions of other people. By shifting your needs from the reliance of others to define you to a simple mutual teamwork exercise of living, you become free.

For example, imagine two players on a soccer team. They pass the ball to each other, but each player has to play the game as they see fit. One player can't kick the ball for the other, and a player can't decide where or when to kick the ball for anyone else. However, the teammates who see no distinction between themselves and others (codependency) are always going to be overly emotional and controlling because they are in fact, out of control. The truth is that no one can control another. The teammate who enjoys the teamwork and respects the other player feels respect within. They simply adapt to situations and are still part of the team but recognize that it is possible to manage their own inner world and feel completely free and full of love—all by themselves.

In a nutshell, the love we all seek has always existed within us and has always been freely available. Popular culture's message that we must behave in a certain manner to earn love is emotionally damaging, and it confuses and undermines many people. In this chapter, we will continue to shed some light on this subtle shift that will lead you to feel more energy, less stress, and more love on a moment-to-moment basis.

Research on Relationships and Health

Research is finally catching up to something we have always known: relationships are important for our health. Maintaining quality relationships not only adds value to our lives but it also leads to less disease and even improves longevity. Research shows that seniors even into their eighties are happier and feel healthier when they maintain quality relationships,[20] while numerous studies show that people who experience chronic loneliness or the absence of close relationships have a greater risk of disease, including coronary heart disease and heart attack. In fact, loneliness may represent a greater threat to public health than obesity.[21]

How does this work? One way is that a lack of relationships can lead to depression, which affects physical health and wellness. Depression slows down our ability to heal from physical illness. It decreases motivation and therefore decreases the engagement of healthy lifestyle choices. Anyone who has felt low—and hasn't everyone?—let alone clinically depressed, knows that energy levels drop and healthy living checklists remain unchecked. If you are feeling low, have a support system to encourage you to receive assistance as needed.

Relationships also affect physical health directly; suppressed emotions and lack of closeness tend to lead to a suppressed immune system, which increases mortality.[22] Imagine the immune system as a big team of security guards dedicated to keeping your body safe from all sorts of threats. If the

20. Robert J. Waldinger and Marc S. Schulz, "What's Love Got to Do with It?: Social Functioning, Perceived Health, and Daily Happiness in Married Octogenarians," *Psychology and Aging* 25(2): 422–431. Jun 2010.

21. "So Lonely I Could Die," *American Psychological Association*. August 2017. http://www.apa.org/news/press/releases/2017/08/lonely-die.aspx.

22. Jorge Daruna, *Introduction to Psychoneuroimmunology*. Waltham, MA: Academic Press, 2004.

head of the team is feeling down and confused, there is chaos among the ranks. Similar things happen in the body and science supports this. When the body is under distress from a health condition or emotional strain, it wears us down over time. The immune system can become weakened, and preexisting conditions overtake our balance.

Luckily there is a great deal we can do to strengthen our relationships and thereby improve our health. Let's start by developing a new understanding of our emotions.

Truths We Experience with Emotions

Emotions and health are linked, and often psychosomatic responses—that is, physical symptoms associated with emotional distress—are the result.

- An upset stomach commonly relates to worry that binds the vagus nerve complex that links the brain and guts.

- A heavy heart grabs the shoulders forward, pulls the neck forward, decreases breathing capacity and reduces the body's function as sadness literally sinks the back into the lungs.

- A pain in the neck is an indication of an underlying annoyance that persists, eventually disrupting sleep and exercise.

- The modern condition known as "text neck" caused by a person using their cell phone or related device while leaning forward has actually caused the spine of many young people to change, increasing the risk for thoracic kyphosis, also known as turtle neck. While this may be considered a solely physical habit, it could also be viewed as a false sense of a connection that leaves a person leaning forward in anticipation of friendship but never achieving it. The person's neck is grasping for an elusive connection but never reaching the goal.

Compared to the vast amount of research on physical ailments, little has been proven about the physical effects of psychosomatic illnesses. However, it's common knowledge that strong emotional states such as sadness, fear, worry, and anger sustained over time are associated with anxiety, depression, and other mental health issues. The effects of strong emotional states on physical health have only been formally researched in recent years, but much has been proven or at least suggested during the short time that this kind of research has been conducted.

Unlike acute medical pains and diseases, psychosomatic imbalances tend to appear in more subtle ways. However, what begins as low levels of stress in the body and mind may lead to anxiety and other health conditions. Learning to understand how to align our relationship beliefs to reality and avoid unnecessary emotional dissonance is where we head next.

Emotions Explained

To understand the yoga view of emotions, start by imagining this scenario: You are reading the news in a crowded airport waiting area, awaiting your flight to be called. From overhead you hear someone being called to the adjacent ticket counter, someone with the same name of your childhood friend. You haven't seen her since her family moved across the country in high school, but it is an unusual name. Could it possibly be her? You look up and there she is. It's been many, many years since you saw one another, but you'd recognize that face anywhere. You walk up and greet her, and the two of you embrace, bursting into simultaneous laughter and tears, exclaiming how much you miss each other's friendship. You know there is little time, so you catch up quickly—locations, kids, jobs. Your friend mentions that her mother recently passed away, you hug her again and update her about your family. You quickly exchange contact information as boarding for her flight is announced.

In this one exchange, you feel a wide range of emotions. There is curiosity at hearing the familiar name, surprise and elation at recognizing your friend. You feel a flash of the loneliness you felt when she moved away back in high school, followed by happiness at how her life has blossomed in the interim, then sadness to hear about her mother's passing, bittersweet memories of how kind her mother had always been to you. Finally, you feel elated again at the thought that you can now have this cherished friend back in your life. As you head back to your seat, a montage of warm memories floods your heart.

Emotions, in a pure definition, are units of mind-body exchange. Something new occurs, and the human mind expresses it as an emotion until the brain has a chance to process and integrate—to accept—the new information. As you review this chance meeting in your mind, the intensity of the emotions subsides. The next time you talk to your friend, you will be happy to hear her voice, but the surprise, elation, and intensity of the sadness will not be there because the information is no longer new. This is the case whether the emotions relate to uplifting situations like this one, or more difficult experiences.

In your brain, the raw emotions contain powerful energy that dissipates as you process new information. But when we don't process our emotions, the energy remains in our minds and bodies and over time can affect our health. This happens especially in situations that challenge us, when things don't happen in the ways we dearly want. If we repress the emotions or simply leave them unacknowledged—that is, when we resist accepting a situation as it is—the unprocessed emotions roil around in our brains and bodies. We develop a pattern of repeating the same emotions, not reaching a place of peace until we process and accept them. Unprocessed emotions add to stress, possibly leading toward disease. Understanding and accepting the roots of our emotions releases that energy, permitting us to see the world in a new way and leaving us in a state of freedom.

What follows may be a novel way for you to think of emotions. Many of us identify with our emotions. When we experience an emotion strongly, we tend to *become* it. "I *am* happy." "I *am* angry." "I *am* afraid." Or, we might bypass our emotions, glossing over them and moving on to the next activity. Both approaches to dealing with emotions can create imbalances that result in other areas of life possibly spiraling out of control. Many unhealthy behaviors not directly related to relationships arise from unprocessed emotions. Overeating, drinking, "retail therapy," and obsessive cleaning can be ways of coping with the pressures of unprocessed emotional energy. By understanding emotions as energies to be processed, we can minimize these impulses and benefit our health in many ways at once. When we adopt the idea that our emotions provide information about how we are responding to the situations we find ourselves in, we can better understand ourselves and our needs in relationships.

Overcoming Obstacles to Relationship Insight

Once you recognize an emotion as information, then you need to process the insight associated with relationships. The *klesas*, or hindrances or distractions to the mind, are a yoga philosophy concept that is helpful for reflecting on our habitual responses in life situations in order to gain insight and create a healthier response. The klesas (different from the koshas, or layers) are ignorance, egoism, attachment, avoidance, and fear. We can trace all of our confused relational responses back to one or more klesas. By understanding the obstacles and recognizing when they are present, we are more likely to be able to overcome them and thus free ourselves from emotional imbalances that affect our relationships. Let's take a look at each hindrance and see how it can be used as a tool for gaining insight into your emotions.

Ignorance or Misunderstanding of Reality

The word "ignorance" in English refers to a lack of knowledge or skill in a worldly sense. But this klesa, called *avidya* in Sanskrit, is spiritual and refers to a misunderstanding of reality. This kind of knowledge is not gained through books or the internet but through introspection, reflection, and wisdom. As said earlier, all the love we seek lies within ourselves and always has. If I believe instead that others are supposed to make me happy, then all of my relationships will be based on that unreal, untrue premise, causing me unnecessary suffering.

When our emotions get the better of us, they color our perception of reality. Oftentimes the emotional charge is so strong that it causes us to completely misunderstand actual reality. The misperceptions happen on several levels at the same time. For example, a driver makes a turn without signaling. The person driving behind him yells at the slowing car and says, "Use your turn signal, you so-and-so!" Now, the first driver didn't know that their turn signal light had just burned out and didn't work. The second driver was upset because he didn't know that the person's light had just broken. Instead, he made a lot of assumptions about the first driver. However, the deeper ignorance was letting another person's driving choices alter his mood. Imagine how this upset driver might treat family members and co-workers. And worse than that, imagine how this person, who has all sorts of expectations of others, feels all day long when people constantly let him down. That is how his "ignorance of reality" clouds his world. By resetting his expectations to a truthful statement like, "I don't control others, I observe and try to be peaceful and compassionate," this same man will find that his day starts with inner peace and it could end that way.

A common cause of ignorance is expectations. We all have expectations about how other people should act and what they should say and do. Our expectations are built around our own experiences and beliefs. When people act in ways that don't align with our expectations, we suffer in many ways.

Objectively, we know that different people do things in different ways. Our expectations reside below our level of consciousness, forming our opinions and desires without our awareness. Conflict can result when another person doesn't measure up, or when we ourselves fall short of a personal expectation. When we hold unrealistic expectations, we set ourselves up for stress and emotional pain. If you find yourself thrown off-kilter by these situations, it helps to examine your expectations and thereby defuse tensions.

Egoism

When we speak of the ego, we tend to think of people who stand out for seeming to always behave as if they are better and more deserving than everyone else. It is easy to identify an egotistic person who, for example, talks about themselves continually, but egoism is not so black-and-white. There are many shades of gray, and an infinite number of distinctions within them that we often are not able to distinguish in ourselves. Notice how you receive compliments or flattery. If you feel proud of yourself due to an accomplishment that was credited to you, does your ego take credit or is there a sense that you are a part of larger processes at work? Does jealousy enter your heart when others succeed? Jealousy and other ego-based thought patterns twist our ego around and cause us misfortune because reality is clouded. If someone else is clever and gifted, it has nothing to do with our particular ego; the fact is that person is gifted. Celebrating others is possible, but the celebration is for the amazing act of nature that created such a person—not for crediting the person's ego.

However, most cultures raise children by bolstering their tiny egos to give them a positive sense of self. This method of praising a child during successes and being silent or punitive during failures causes the child to feel love via performance instead of feeling loved regardless of any external means. Here is an example of building the ego up while associating performance with love: "Johnny, you played great and scored the winning goal! Without you, the team would have lost!" Although it at first sounds positive, the underlying message is "you are a good kid because you scored a goal." Contrast this scene with: "Johnny, I see your team won on your final goal of the game, how did that play develop? What did you learn from that game?" This second reflection is process oriented and doesn't make Johnny feel better than if he would have if he missed the final shot and his team lost. The same approach could apply: "Oh, Johnny, your team lost when you missed the final kick, what did you learn from that miskick? How did that play develop?" Winning or losing has no effect on the love that Johnny's ego may feel, as the love is unrelated to the outcome of the game.

Even an average-sized ego can keep us from seeing the truth about a situation, because we all see things from our own point of view. While in normal circumstances this isn't a problem, if done too often, or to an extreme, it can be detrimental in a relationship. Ego causes us to believe and to insist that we know better, that our way of doing things is superior. It can result in exaggerating the value of our own contributions to the relationship and taking for granted the other person's contributions.

The counterpoint to too much ego is not too little. In fact, perhaps surprisingly, too little can be just as problematic as too much. The person in a relationship who always bends to the other's wishes, who doesn't speak up for his or her own needs, is being dishonest with their partners and themselves. Partners have to feel they can rely on one another and honest exchange is a requirement to build that kind of trust.

Instead, the too-little ego person's solution to the ego obstacle is to gain approval by adopting the other person's point of view. For example, if I agree with everything my spouse says, I may be trying to keep harmony by denying my personal opinion. By displaying no ego, the passive person is habitually telling small lies, or worse, setting themselves up to eventually explode when the loss of self becomes deafening.

The answer then is a balanced ego, one that takes everyone's needs and feelings into account.

EXERCISE How Much Ego Is in Your World?

Consider the following questions.

- Are you a person with too much or too little ego?

- Or, does your ego revolve around the situation? Do you behave one way at work and another way at home?

- How does your upbringing effect the way your ego functions?

- How do you listen to others? If you are a dominant person, do you listen to others or are you asserting your viewpoint constantly, as a way to feel comfortable?

- On the contrary, if you are passive, are you listening to everything without saying anything?

- Are you capable of completely listening to another person without judgment and remain balanced?

Attachment

In our culture, attachment can mean love. The meaning here is different. Attachment in yoga is when our desire to hold close to someone or something is so strong that an intense form of grasping for the external thing occurs. Like with ego, smaller, more mundane versions of attachments can also cause problems. For example, we have a belief, an idea, or a way of doing things that has perhaps outlived its usefulness, but we grasp onto it like to an invisible security blanket, holding on beyond the point of reason. "I need you to act like this for me to be happy, I need you to do this task so I can be happy," are examples of attachments.

Let's look at the concept of attachment a little more closely. In yoga, attachment is defined as the confusion between the higher self and the pleasures of the senses. The desire for water (thirst) is a healthy craving. Our modern materialistic consumer culture equates a successful life with the accumulation of material possessions, power, and external beauty. Suffering happens when we think that the "pleasurable" thing will bring us long-term happiness; attachments to passing fancies will inevitably lead to pain. Drinking some water is a realistic need for life, but the external comforts are an illusion.

Often, the fuel of attachment is discomfort or perceived pain. In this light, anything from drugs to shopping can be used in an attempt to distract ourselves. Yet we all know that once the party is over or the new shoes get scuffed, the pain persists, and we are still left to face ourselves. It is here we have a choice to break the cycle by becoming willing to accept life and seek out support systems to help us cope and eventually heal.

During youth, a person gifted with material resources and good health can survive for a while in an illusion of material happiness. However, as that person ages, various problems occur that cannot be solved no matter the strength or conviction of the person's belief in materialism. Loved ones pass away, children have problems, money is lost, and health declines as we age. By gradually recognizing and releasing our attachments to external forms of happiness, we learn to find happiness from within. Through focusing on the larger reality, one learns that true peace is of a spiritual nature.

Positive forms of attachment do exist. Any form of mild attachment that edifies or increases one's spiritual sense is considered beneficial. Attachment to family members occurs and fosters one's ability to love unconditionally. While it is painful when a family member leaves or dies, the attachment ultimately teaches a person to reduce their ego, overcome selfishness, and grow in faith. Attachment to God or religious faith or seeking the spiritual may also cause purification as benevolent action can help us to expand our consciousness. Positive attachment in these cases depends on a healthy attitude, including not controlling others or depending on them for personal happiness. Likewise, a healthy connection to one's religion will never attempt to negate others' belief systems.

When a relationship with a loved one or to a religion or spiritual path becomes possessive, it no longer has a positive effect. The rigid adherence to one's religion—yes, even a rigid belief in yoga practices or certain ways of living—can turn a positive attachment into a destructive obsession. Possession in relationships implies that the possessor's happiness is reliant on the other person. These positive attachments may assist spiritual growth at first but are not pure; with faith and practice even positive attachments will diminish as one realizes the difference between love and appreciation, and attachment.

The solution for these kinds of attachments is first to become aware of them, then to let them go, or modify them to a form that is better suited to our current situation. Freed from our inflexible positions, we can view each new situation with fresh eyes and a clear head. Finding our feelings of faith and trust gives us the courage we need to let go. Often after releasing an attachment, we look back and wonder why we were so reluctant to let it go.

EXERCISE Releasing Attachments

1. Make a list of your prized possessions, those things you won that mean the most to you. Ask yourself a sincere question: Could you do without these items? While there is no need to give away possessions, examine whether or not you are able to release your attachment to these things. Look at where your happiness comes from.

2. Pick one of the items and practice the exercise by drawing a circle around your attachment. Accept the attachment by looking deeper into the situation and begin to understand the spiritual essence of what you are seeking from the material thing. What does that item represent to you?

3. Make a list of your beliefs about relationships. How are you attached to your ideas as being superior to other belief systems? Attempt to honor the beliefs of others as a method to release the traces of possession of a relationship.

Avoidance

On the flip side of attachments are aversions, which make our world smaller. They cause us to miss out on people, things, experiences, or ideas without really understanding why, based usually on strong, gut-level feelings of anger or disgust. (Anxiety has the same effects but is caused by fear, which we'll discuss later.) In relationships, avoidance causes issues in various ways. People who avoid confrontation don't have a chance to work out differences. Those who avoid new experiences or ideas may frustrate their more adventurous partners, leading to relationship issues small and large.

Aversion can be particularly tricky to work with, as it can manifest as anger (a defense mechanism), discontent, denial, avoidance, and procrastination. All these behaviors can cause severe disruptions in relationships. When a situation is at the foreground of our awareness, we are likely to relive our negative emotions over and over again. In other words, it is common to dwell

133

on a situation that is disagreeable to one person. But situations in and of themselves are neutral; therefore, the emotion is simply showing the roots of aversion. Take for example a pile of trash dumped in a public park. Most people detest litter, especially where children might play. But the onlooker's anger is simply a representation of his or her views about litter. The story is colored by the person's views on litter. Little did anyone realize that the pile of trash was one of twenty that the local community organization was in the process of clearing after last night's huge party for the neighborhood children where five hundred people joined together to hear a famous storyteller entertain children and parents alike.

An even more subtle expression is an aversion to one's own personality, which shows up as negative self-talk or excessive self-criticism. This type of behavior exists in people who easily accept the shortcomings of others but are not able to accept their own unique set of challenges. Forms of this kind of aversion usually relate to one's appearance, body shape, cultural or professional status, or failure regarding self-imposed expectations in life.

More difficult, perhaps, are our aversions to the people in our lives, or events we perceive to be unjust, immoral, or harmful. When we are angry with someone, we are suffering from aversion. Typically when we find something about someone else that we have a strong aversion to, we are usually projecting. This means that we see qualities that we do not like about ourselves in others. Or we might see others in the present as someone else who harmed us a long time ago or arouses our vulnerabilities in some other way. In these situations, people we dislike can actually become our greatest teachers. When we learn the truth about our interpretation and learn to love and accept the person who challenges us, what we're actually doing is learning to love ourselves and heal the past. An aversion, like an attachment, is a self-constructed false view of reality. When we have this kind of aversion to a person or event, we are looking with our own biases in a way that is really an error on our part.

Just like healthy fears, healthy aversions can help us to avoid danger or undo pain. Unhealthy aversions reduce the feeling of love. Aversion prevents us from facing a situation within ourselves or from addressing a situation with another. As a hidden thought, aversion harms. Once expressed, it can be understood, accepted, and transformed.

Identifying our aversions and forming a resolve to overcome them is the vehicle for moving past them. Like attachments, aversions are fed by insecurities. Building trust and faith propel the process forward.

EXERCISE Admitting Your Avoidances Have No Power

This exercise comes in two parts. Part 1 asks you to look at aversions in general. Part 2 specifically refers to an aversion in a relationship.

Part 1

1. Make a list of things you dislike. Include chores, people, difficult situations, and anything you dread.

2. Distinguish two categories in the list, things that harm you and things that are neutral. Washing the dishes is neutral, while passing a dangerous area at night is potentially dangerous.

3. Understand how the activity you dread is really neutral, even while some sort of discomfort may be involved.

4. Examine your resistance to the activity. Where do you think it comes from? Do you feel threatened or vulnerable in some way, even if it is not dangerous? Does it remind you of a time in your past when you felt threatened or vulnerable? Might it remind you of something about yourself that you dislike?

5. Find creative ways to participate in neutral activities without any mental disturbance. Release your resistance to the activity. Once you do, notice how much stress a negative attitude absorbs and how you feel after you have released that stress.

Part 2

1. Identify one specific aversion within the context of a current relationship.

2. Relate this aversion to a prior pain, hurt, or discomfort, asking yourself the same questions as in part 1.

3. Taking the role of witness or compassionate observer, attempt to understand this pain, hurt, or discomfort by feeling it.

4. Trace this feeling's roots to a thought pattern that allows you to be vulnerable to this pain or hurt.

5. Now devise a more self-reliant perspective to handle this situation from a point of stability instead of weakness.

6. Note that this step will be difficult, especially if the aversion is deep in your personality or past. Seeking assistance from a professional or a compassionate friend can be helpful.

Fear

Fear is an essential emotion, signaling us when we are in danger. Our fears can also become exaggerated, causing us to react strongly in situations that are objectively safe. Phobias about things such as darkness, benign insects, or crowds fit this description as fears greatly magnify minor risks.

Fear in the context of a relationship signals us about threats to our emotional safety. It centers on anticipation of change and loss: Will our marriage or partnership survive the challenges that life directs at it? What will happen to our relationships with our parents as they age or our children as they grow up? Will a friendship persist despite a serious argument? Like phobias, fears about relationships sometimes alert us to true jeopardy but are more often about our self-doubts. Living with too much fear concerning relationships diminishes the love, joy, and comfort they are meant to provide.

Most of us have a pattern at the core of our fears around relationship loss, usually rooted in our early lives, perhaps related to abandonment or neglect. Some might have a deep-seated fear of conflict. Others might fear being given more responsibility than they can handle, or having their autonomy taken away. Some fear physical harm. Beyond the scope of primal safety, unnecessary fear creates stress. Many parts of our society use fear as a motivational force. "If you don't work hard, you will not be successful. Do your homework or you will be unhappy in your future." But think how beneficial it is when these motivations are accomplished by positive means. "Study to learn and be happy. Work hard because your work helps others!" When looking at these positive versus negative approaches, it is easy to see that positive motivations create positive results, without the need to activate the human fight or flight system to produce excellence.

Living with fear is not total living. A preoccupation with worry over the future removes you from the present. If your mind is not here in each moment, you are missing out on life. Thus, fear distracts us from living fully. In yoga we learn that understanding the depths of our fears helps us live in a liberated fashion. As we uncover our patterns, we can begin to accept the fears head on and eventually feel courageous, because courage is the acceptance of fear.

EXERCISE Identifying Fears

This also comes in two parts, one for general fears and one in terms of a relationship.

Part 1

1. Make a list of all the things you fear. As you do this, examine things that may be very subtle. Fears of your work review, parental approval, neighbors' opinions, your future, and even minor worries count.

2. As you review this list, step back from it to gain a larger perspective. Accept the feelings of fear and remain aware of the fear. Think deeply on distant fears, allowing you to possibly uncover issues below the surface.

3. Examine if these fears motivate you to work too hard or to behave in an unhealthy way. You can evaluate your motivations behind actions and understand the sources of these evaluations.

4. Now, align the situation with positive qualities.

Part 2

1. As you begin to see the bigger picture of your fears and motivations, relate them to a current relationship.

2. Spend some time journaling on how fear affects your actions and choices in the relationship dynamic.

3. As you accept these fears, visualize the courageous you interacting as your true self in the relationship.

A Tool for Processing Emotional Insights

Now that you have an awareness of the hindrances or blocks that create stress responses, you can use this section to help you access additional insights into your emotions and relationships. As you have been learning in this chapter, giving time and attention to your relationship motives is an important aspect in self-understanding that helps you to uncover deep, unconscious patterns. In understanding those patterns, you can begin to see how emotions reveal deeper aspects of ourselves and, what's more, how those patterns affect relationships and create stress. Use the following four questions for processing your emotional insights.

1. **What is the story I am telling myself?** As humans, we regularly create stories in our minds to make sense of our world. When a new situation causes our emotions to run high, our stories reflect that fact. We weave the stories from an emotional point of view. Notice what your story is and where in the story your emotions take hold the strongest.

2. **What am I feeling?** Emotions fuel our stories, but that doesn't mean we are consciously aware of them or even know which ones they are. Let go of what you are thinking and focus on your feelings. What emotions do you feel? Can you name them?

3. **Where am I feeling it?** Emotional energy makes itself felt as tension in the body. Do a body scan and notice where you feel tight. Joints—especially shoulders, hips, and the jaw—are a common place for emotions to be held. Headaches and upset stomachs are other frequent manifestations of emotion. So are feelings of tightness around the throat, heart, and lower back. Do you experience tension in any of those places? Somewhere else?

4. **Is there a past experience or event that relates to the current situation in my life?** When we harbor unacknowledged or repressed emotions, they may emerge at inappropriate times. If you find that your emotional reaction to a new situation is ill-fitted or out of proportion, it could be an indication of old emotional energy emerging. Use that insight as a jumping-off point for self-reflection.

EXERCISE Your Personalized Plan for
Building Strong Relationships

After a number of powerful exercises in this chapter, please notice which exercise gripped you the most. Spend more time on this exercise to derive additional insights.

1. Perhaps you can use this new perspective to inspire you to find some support on this issue.

2. Plan a few steps to follow regarding any insights this chapter has helped you assess. Recognizing the connection that relationships have to your health allows you to continue this journey through each and every aspect of your overall healthy lifestyle.

Chapter Summary

In this chapter, we explored how high-quality relationships enrich our lives with love, support, companionship and joy, and reinforce our health. Studies show a direct link between our relationships and the quality of our physical and mental health. We also explored the body-mind connection between our emotion, in addition to how unprocessed emotions affect the physical body and our relationship with self and others.

The klesas, or hindrances of the mind were introduced as tools for reflecting on and gaining insight from our emotional responses. The five klesas are:

• Ignorance: Misunderstanding reality, rather than an absence of knowledge. The root of all klesas, ignorance colors our perception of reality and triggers emotional responses and behaviors that often create conflict in relationships.

• Egoism: Both excess egos and diminished egos can affects relationships adversely. Balanced egos consider the welfare of all parties.

• Attachment: Over-attachment or possessiveness occurs when a person's happiness is dependent on another. This creates unrealistic expectations and demands on others and unnecessary conflict within the relationship. It also leaves the attached person feeling anxious because their happiness depends on things outside their control.

- Avoidance: Showing up in many forms in relationships, avoidance prevents us from fully connecting to others, and from fully experiencing life. It creates a disconnect within the relationship.
- Fear: Unhealthy fear drives our behaviors within a relationship, causing us to act from a place of worry and anxiety, making it impossible to be fully present with others.

Through exercises designed to build awareness about hindrances of the mind and how they impact your emotions, behaviors and relationships, you began to shift from unconscious habits and patterns. You gained conscious awareness and, through practice, learned to shift into healthier and more effective behaviors within your relationships.

In the next chapter, we consider our relationship to the natural world—the great outdoors! We also explore the spaces where we live and how those spaces effect our health.

eight
HARNESSING THE
POWER OF THE
NATURAL WORLD

Nature offers us a sense of perspective. Looking out at the horizon over the ocean, gazing up at a towering pine tree or at the night sky inspires a sense of awe. The majesty of the natural world reassures us that we and every living thing on the planet are connected to something greater than ourselves. The yogic path of the intellect, or jnana, relates to our ability to recognize this bigger picture of connection that the natural world inspires. As we spend time in nature and embrace this bigger picture of connection, we feel a sense of peace and harmony. Our eyes are opened to the innate gifts of the natural world that support our health.

Similarly, the environments in which we spend time, e.g., home or work, and the characteristics associated with them—space, light, noise, colors, energy, and so on—affect our health. Our nervous systems are constantly adjusting to environmental stimuli. Some are calming while others create agitation. How we function in the spaces we move in and out of daily directly affects stress and anxiety levels, which carry over into our attitudes about all other areas of our lives. Spending time in nature and harnessing the power of its qualities to benefit health helps balance out the intense stimulation of modern-day life.

In this chapter, we focus on the natural world as a natural health source. Like the previous chapters, the exercises and practices guide you to new insights and help you create a plan to incorporate new, healthful habits in your life.

The Natural World and Your Health

Over the last several decades, technological advances have transformed everyday life. Home computers entered the market in 1977 and laptop use took off during the 1990s. Apple first released the iPhone in 2007. Scientists don't yet know all the ways technology influences our health *or* the health of our planet, but we do know that mental health disorders are increasing and technology is one of the reasons.

At the same time, surely as a result, people began spending significantly more time indoors. Twenty-first-century Americans spend on average about 87 percent of their time indoors, plus another 6 percent enclosed in cars, a far cry from most of our grandparents. Obesity, attention disorders, anxiety, and depression may all be attributed to a lack of nature.

As these new health issues arose so did the idea of *biophilia,* or love of the living world. This belief states that because humans evolved within nature, we have a biological need to connect with it; when we don't, our health suffers. A new and growing field of research led by Japanese scientists proves that idea is true. "Forest Bathing," or spending time "soaking in" nature, has been shown to reduce stress; strengthen the immune and cardiovascular systems; boost energy, mood, creativity, and concentration; and even increase length of life.

It is more important now than ever to engage with the outdoors. The more high-tech we become, the more we need to spend time in nature.

EXERCISE Your Nature and Health Baseline

Take out your journal and spend some time reflecting on your current relationship with nature. Remember to do your best to remain open minded and non-judgmental. This process is designed to help you objectively see where you are and where you may want to go from here. Consider the following questions:

- On an average week, how much time do you spend outside in natural surroundings?
- What types of places do you frequent? Which natural spaces are your favorite and why?
- When you are in nature, what are you doing?
  - Are you involved in some form of activity? If so, which ones are your favorites?
  - Do you actively connect with your surroundings? Or are they simply a background for your activities?
  - Do you bring your phone or other devices with you? If so, how much are you using them during your time outside?
- What motivates you to be outside?
- What limits your time outside?
- Describe the benefits you receive from your time in nature. Reflect on the different aspects of your life
- Do you feel you have enough time out in nature, or would you benefit from more time?

Take a look through your responses and see where you may want to make adjustments. Perhaps you would like more time outdoors. Maybe you are longing to increase the quality of your connection with nature. Or perhaps you wish to engage in new or different activities while in nature. On a clean page in your journal, brainstorm some creative ways to make these changes where desired. Consider incorporating the other lifestyle areas of this book (movement, relationships, rest, and so forth) into your outdoor time. Keep these reflections available to turn back to later in this chapter.

Nature's Natural Health Qualities

The scientific research that supports the need for nature in our lives rests on the abundant healthful qualities the natural world supplies. Science looks to the chemicals found in nature and we are in the infancy of studying this sort of phenomena. Trees emit phytoncides, molecules that give off their distinctive scents. These substances protect the trees and also contain healing powers for humans, as they can be distilled into essential oils with properties that fight against bacteria, microbes, and even fungi that can affect human health. Even the dirt found in forests provides beneficial properties. In cities, trees serve a critical filtering purpose, filtering out air pollution that we humans inhale into our lungs.[23] (Yes, it's important to note that nature found in cities counts too! You don't have to go deep into a forest to enjoy the health benefits.)

Different qualities in the air around us affect health as well. Have you ever wondered why the air near the beach, mountains, or waterfalls feels so much cleaner and healthier than the air around dust, humidity, and pollution? Clean, healthy air is rich in negative ions that bond with common pollutants and allergens and cause them to drop down toward the ground, away from the air we breathe. The effect is so dramatic that science shows people who spend more time in clean, negatively charged air are less likely to experience depression and may have better mood, reduced anxiety, and improved sleep.[24]

Positive ions, on the other hand, are noted in great quantities during high winds, humidity, and just before electrical storms. They've been shown to cause fatigue and a host of related symptoms. These ions are also associated with artificial environments; areas around clothes dryers, photocopiers, printers, and florescent lighting are positive ion hot spots. Since not many of us can spend all of our time near waterfalls and away from printers, we need to restore balance to our living environments in ways that cause us to feel uplifted. Examine new technological advances from a health standpoint as well as convenience when deciding what you want in your home.

Getting the Most Out of Natural World Experiences

To make the most of natural experiences, we need to attend to them using our senses to drink in the natural surroundings of the woods or a city park. As a society, we're surprisingly out of practice at using our senses. Our eyes

23. Qing Li, *Forest Bathing: How Trees Can Help You Find Health and Happiness*, New York: Viking, 2018.

24. Vanessa Perez, Dominik D. Alexander, William H. Bailey, "Air Ions and Mood Outcomes: A Review and Meta-analysis", *BMC Psychiatry* 13: 29. 2013. https://www.ncbi.nlm.nih.gov /pmc/articles/PMC3598548/.

are accustomed to flat screens close to our faces, our fingers to the blank feel of plastic. We're used to such high levels of noise that many of us are uncomfortable in nature's relative silence.

Instead, we want to adopt the attitude of forest bathing, the point of which is to be mindful and present in nature, not to "do" or achieve anything with nature as a backdrop. Our cultural preference for achieving something, meeting a goal, doing something we can measure, may also get in our way of paying attention to the natural world. Running or getting in our ten thousand steps outdoors is wonderful but has a different spirit. Obviously, forest bathing is easier if you are unplugged; if you find the idea challenging, you can wean yourself from technology slowly, perhaps turning off your cell phone for five minutes in the woods to start and building up to longer. Or take the rip-off-the-bandage approach and leave it home!

So then what should you be doing? When in nature, even in a city park, try closing your eyes and focusing on the sounds and the different fragrances of the various plants and trees. When your eyes are open, look for the beauty of nature's patterns—branches, spirals, spokes. Yogic breathing exercises or meditation techniques are perfect to help you slow down and be where you are in time and space, allowing you to more fully appreciate the experience.

It even helps to take your shoes off. Just as electrical work has to be grounded, human beings feel more balanced and centered when in direct contact with the earth's healing electro-magnetic force. (Traditional shoes made of natural materials conducted this force into earlier humans' feet, but rubber-soled shoes do not.) Walking barefoot on the beach is perfect for this. Once you begin to let nature into your being through your senses, you might find that its wisdom transforms your outlook. Be creative when thinking how to connect to nature.

If you're already a yoga practitioner, you know that poses are another way to give a great sense of grounding and feeling to your body, a complete ecosystem in and of itself. When doing yoga on your own or in a class, feel all the aspects of your body and mind, much like you would a forest. Notice your feet and body connecting to the earth like tree roots or rocks in the soil. Feel your skin as if it were the leaves soaking in sunlight. Your breath is like the wind and fresh air. Your blood pulses through your body as streams that flow down hillsides. Your muscles are like the movement of new saplings, or of animals that move or fish that swim. Use the opportunity to notice all aspects of your senses. Then remember those feelings and sensations during other times of your daily life.

With a little creativity, you will find plenty of ways to further connect to nature. Consider the following ideas:

- Dine outside when the weather is nice.
- Plant a small garden or create a pot garden on your balcony.
- Take a blanket or chair to the local park to read a book or have a picnic with friends or family.
- Go for a short walk outside during your lunch breaks.
- Visit local wildlife preserves, arboretums, and other nature sanctuaries.
- When outside, breathe in the air. Take in the sights and sounds and smells of nature.
- Notice the feel of the sun and air on your skin.
- Consciously feel your feet as you walk on the ground, sensing gravity, feeling connected to the earth.
- Learn about local wildlife and plants. You could make a game of identifying them when you are out; if you have kids, you can do this together.
- Sit outside and identify shapes you see in the clouds.
- Meditate under a tree, in a field, or along a stream.
- Stargaze.
- Go to local farm stands and farmers markets to get fresh, local food. Find creative activities to do with kids if you have them, like making bird feeders and hanging them near a window or porch and watching who comes to visit. Skip rocks. Forage for leaves, acorns, and pine cones and make arts and crafts with them. Make daisy or dandelion chains.

Bringing the Natural World Indoors

Bringing more of nature indoors helps to re-create the sense of peace and harmony you enjoy outdoors. Here are a few ideas for ways to accomplish this, using the essential elements of earth, fire, water, and air as a guide.

Earth

Choose natural materials to fill your home—wooden furniture, wood or ceramic kitchenware, rugs and linens made from natural fibers. Here are more suggestions:

- Decorate with wood, stone, and glass.
- Make liberal use of indoor greenery.
- Consider bird feeders, or plant flowers outdoors that attract bees, butterflies, or hummingbirds.
- If it fits your lifestyle, get a pet.

Fire

Heat has the power to release the transforming scents of nature inside your home. Here are a few suggestions for how to harness the power of fire:

- Cook fresh food using fragrant herbs and spices.
- Use a diffuser or other device with essential oils. If you like, burn incense, although be aware that the smoke from incense can be an irritant for some.[25]
- Especially in winter, strings of "fairy lights" and candles create warm, welcoming light. Many people prefer soy wax or beeswax candles over paraffin, which is a petroleum-based product. Be sure there is plenty of ventilation around a burning candle. Parents of young children and some pet owners have to weigh safety risks.[26]

Water

Water is readily available in our homes, so it's easy to overlook its wonder. Here are some suggestions for better using and appreciating it:

---

25. National Health Services, "Is Incense Smoke More Dangerous than Tobacco Smoke?" August 2015. https://www.nhs.uk/news/cancer/is-incense-smoke-more-dangerous-than-tobacco-smoke/.

26. EPA Office of Research and Development. "Candles and Incense as Potential Sources of Indoor Air Pollution: Market Analysis and Literature Review," January 2001. https://nepis.epa.gov/Adobe/PDF/P1009BZL.pdf.

- Never underestimate the power of water as a cleanser. Often it may be all you need, allowing you to avoid harsher chemicals.

- Learn about your local water source.

- Look into the safety of your drinking water and decide if you need a filtration system. Finding out if your water is particularly hard or soft allows you to make adjustments, if necessary, to maximize cleaning power and minimize possible damage to your pipes.

- Ritualize your daily hygiene practices to bring consciousness to how water supports your body.

- Be mindful from time to time of the great gift that is indoor plumbing.

Air

Industrial areas, inner cities near highways, and places where coal is used for energy are obvious areas of outdoor pollution. However, modern life has altered the indoor air that humans breathe in many ways, though you might not notice because indoor air pollution can be odorless and invisible. In some instances, it's even possible for indoor air pollution to pose a greater health risk than outdoor air pollution. Much of the modern person's living and working conditions are comfortable in terms of temperature, but that means sealing up spaces against air flow to keep the temperature near 70 degrees in winter and summer. Using air conditioning requires windows to be shut and air leaks sealed. It's a commonplace habit to keep office windows and home windows closed nearly all year. Imagine how different that is from people who live closer to nature! If you are a person used to outdoor living, you will immediately notice stagnant indoor air; it will smell unpleasant. Try a few of these interventions to bring in fresh air to your living spaces.

- Open a window daily! Fresh air moves and purifies stale indoor air. Keep this in mind even during cold winter months, or if your house is closed up for air conditioning.

- Smell outdoor air the way a sommelier appreciates the aroma of wine. Smell the changes in air from low to high pressure and with the changes in the seasons.

- Become accustomed to outdoor air so you can detect when to air out your home.
- Clean thoroughly to control dust, mold, and other irritants.
- Keep air circulated by area fans when cooling is necessary.
- Use indoor plants to clean your air. Indoor plants offer oxygen and remove harmful compounds.
- If you have an interest in essential oils, enjoy diffusers or other forms of scenting your home.
- In dry climates (or dry indoor climates due to heating or air conditioning), make sure there is enough moisture in your air.

Products and Environmental Safety

A few hundred years ago, everything inside a home from furniture to cleaning materials to skin lotions was made from natural materials. There simply wasn't any other option. Now of course many items are synthetic. New products have transformed our lives but also create hazards that can negatively impact our health. When they do, it's known as environmental illness, meaning that the environment played a significant role in producing physical symptoms. Allergies to products such as latex are a very common example of environmental illness. Headaches caused by product fumes is another example. Kerosene heaters, leaks from furnaces and chimneys, exhaust from cars, tobacco smoke, and household products like paint strippers, aerosol sprays and even products sold as air fresheners are among many other culprits that can contribute to environmental illness indoors.[27] (None of this means to lessen the risk of outdoor pollution on health! In one of many examples, research shows clearly that outdoor air pollution in urban areas causes asthma symptoms to worsen.[28])

Unfortunately, trying to gather reliable information about product safety is frustratingly difficult. In the United States as this book is being written, we know a great deal about the foods we eat and drink and the medications

27. US Environmental Protection Agency, "The Inside Story: A Guide to Indoor Air Quality," https://www.epa.gov/indoor-air-quality-iaq/inside-story-guide-indoor-air-quality.

28. Michael Guarnieri and John R. Balmes, "Outdoor Air Pollution and Asthma" Lancet 383 (9928): 1581–1592. May 3, 2014. doi: 10.1016/S0140-6736(14)60617-6.

we take thanks to the Food and Drug Administration (FDA), which regulates these items. But the FDA has far less power over other types of products. The Environmental Protection Agency (EPA) collects information every four years about chemicals produced in large quantities, and it requires manufacturers to list ingredients that are recognized as potentially harmful. Regulations have led to warning labels on certain products but, unlike groceries, no ingredient lists.

While a lack of information does not necessarily indicate a product is harmful, many people wish for more information about the products they buy. After all, food and drugs are regulated because we ingest them, but there are other routes for products to enter our bodies. We inhale fumes from the air into our lungs. Our skin absorbs whatever types of lotions, creams, or oils we apply. In the relative information vacuum, organizations have emerged that monitor ingredients and track product safety, and individuals publish information online. You might have favorite sites you consult. Unfortunately, controversy abounds; some information sources do a great deal of research, while some publish speculation as fact. Some of the organizations enjoy a good measure of public trust, even while scientists accuse them of inaccuracy and bias.

On the commercial side, some consumers believe in the power of the market to influence manufacturers' behavior. They say it's in the best interest of companies to create safe, effective products because doing otherwise would be terrible for business. Other people believe that the companies' economic self-interest makes them inherently suspect.

With so many unanswered questions and bad precedents, it's no wonder many of us choose a "better safe than sorry" approach. We may choose products that contain only natural ingredients that are clearly listed on a label from companies that freely publish information about what they use and how it works. We may seek out individual artisans at craft fairs or online and converse with them directly about their products. We learn to use simple, natural methods to accomplish what we need to do in our homes and on our bodies, or even make our own products.

Following are a few natural substitutions you can make to keep yourself and your home clean, that don't require additional effort.

- **Mouthwash**. Rinsing with saltwater kills the germs that contribute to bad breath and helps reduce any mouth swelling. Many commercial mouthwashes, on the other hand, contain large amounts of alcohol that can cause irritation and dry mouth, which ironically can contribute to mouth odor.

- **Moisturizer.** Oils from coconuts and sesame seeds make excellent skin moisturizers without adding chemicals or dyes. This is important because the skin absorbs whatever materials are rubbed into it. Simply rub the oil over your skin just after a shower.

- **Cleaner.** White vinegar makes an excellent all-purpose cleaner for countertops, chrome, and windows. The smell is strong but not any more than many chemical cleaners. Use it diluted with water for general use, and straight to remove stains.

- **Natural Freshener.** Notice what products you might be able to simply do without. Dryer sheets are popular but completely optional, and on a sunny day with a clothesline, so are dryers. Make use of fresh air instead of sprays for odor problems. Wash kitchen trash containers and leave them outdoors overnight periodically to relieve odor buildup; baking soda is also a wonderful kitchen or bathroom deodorant. To freshen a smelly bedroom, just cleaning up, doing laundry, and opening a window works better than chemical sprays.

- **Personal Care.** Follow the same thought process with personal care products. Nail polish and remover contain harsh chemicals. Can you do without? If you don't sweat heavily, maybe you can forgo underarm products, especially in cooler weather. If that doesn't work for you, substitute a natural deodorant instead of an antiperspirant. Deodorants are safer as they affect odor without blocking the body's natural sweating process. Antiperspirants use volatile compounds that thwart the body's ability to cleanse from within.

To Use or Not to Use?

In some cases, we do know what the ingredients are in our personal care products but don't know if they are safe. The trouble is that experts don't agree. A primary example is toothpaste. Should we definitely choose one with fluoride to fight cavities, or one without? The American Dental Association, the nation's largest professional group for dentists, stands firmly behind fluoride as a proven, effective means of reducing cavities and even reversing the beginnings of tooth decay.[29] Experts point to water fluoridation as a great victory in public health, providing an equitable, cost-effective dental health boon to all members of most communities, regardless of age or socioeconomic status.[30]

In opposition stands the International Academy of Oral Medicine and Toxicology (IAOMT), a smaller organization of dental professionals who promote biological dentistry, an approach that seeks the safest, least toxic way to accomplish the goals of modern dentistry. They believe exposure to fluoride poses a serious health risk. They point out that human exposure to fluoride has increased dramatically since water fluoridation began in the 1940s, and that different people, including infants, children, and diabetics, are more severely and adversely affected by fluoridation. The IAOMT advocates for working toward eliminating it from avoidable sources, including toothpaste.[31]

Sunscreen is another controversy. There's no reasonable doubt that it reduces the risk of skin cancer. But it also stands in the way of the body's natural production of vitamin D and may be harmful to the balance of marine life in our oceans.

Does the uncertainty and confusion cause you stress? If so, you're certainly not alone. It may help to remember that all decisions are individual. Some people are more sensitive to some chemicals than others. One person may be severely affected by a particular substance while another appears to tolerate it without difficulty. If you are allergic to plants or trees, you know that even natural products can be safe for most people and problematic for others. Genetic conditions and predisposition to disease is another factor

---

29. American Dental Association, "Oral Health Topics: Toothpastes," https://www.ada.org/en /member-center/oral-health-topics/toothpastes.

30. Centers for Disease Control and Prevention, "Achievements in Public Health, 1900–1999: Fluoridation of Drinking Water to Prevent Dental Caries," https://www.cdc.gov/mmwr /preview/mmwrhtml/mm4841a1.htm.

31. International Academy of Oral Medicine and Technology, "The IAOMT is concerned about the many sources of fluoride and health risks from this exposure," https://iaomt .org/resources/fluoride-facts/.

to consider. If you are prone to skin cancer due to genetics or climate, you might err on the side of more sunscreen use.

Also remember that the decisions about the products you use in your house and for personal care are but one piece of your overall health picture. Glance at the other chapters in this book. Do you get regular exercise? Eat reasonably well? Make efforts to manage your stress? Walk in the woods periodically? If you practice a healthy lifestyle—it doesn't have to be perfect, but good—you are giving a huge, healthy head start to yourself and your family. You can't control everything; you can only do what you can do. The best bottom-line advice is to do the best you can to live in tune with nature but *without* getting yourself too worked up. Agitation leads to the stress that we are trying to minimize!

Suggestions for Green Living

Due to the powerful relationship between the natural world and health, it is vital for us to continue caring for the natural spaces still available on our planet. As you set goals to improve your health, consider the health of the planet as well. The success of the one depends in many ways on the success of the other. Consider the following suggestions to incorporate green living into your lifestyle and comprehensive health plan.

- Research renewable energy sources in your area and implement one of these sources in your home.
- Consider using more fuel-efficient transportation options.
- Look for small ways to conserve resources within your home. Turn your thermostat down a little in winter and up a little in summer; and turn off the water while you brush your teeth. Small changes add up to significant impact.
- Ask that all family members practice "reduce, reuse, recycle" with an emphasis on "reduce," especially for synthetic substances like plastic.
- Eat locally sourced food when possible and make more of your food choices from lower on the food chain. Relying more on a plant-based diet can benefit the environment and decreases reliance on packaged, processed foods.

- Maximize native plants in your yard. Look into the no-mow movement to transform grass lawns into more natural alternatives, which reduce the perceived need for harmful herbicides and frequent watering.

- Cease using any chemicals on outdoor spaces as those same chemicals kill wildlife and wild plants and pollute our water, yet they represent big business. Our culture tells us that a perfectly green lawn is the ultimate outdoor goal. If this is true for you, it might be necessary to shift your perspective so that the goal becomes creating and preserving a working ecosystem.

- Plant trees. They conserve water by drawing rain into the ground via their roots and provide homes and sustenance for wildlife. And as mentioned in the section on forest bathing, they have multiple health benefits for humans.

- Reduce or eliminate single-use plastics and only use BPA-free plastics.

EXERCISE Your Personalized Plan for Creating Healthy Environments Indoors and Outdoors

Throughout this chapter, you've received a variety of suggestions and practices to create a deeper connection with the natural world. Next, develop a plan to incorporate these into your self-care routine.

Listen

Reflect back to the journal entry you created at the beginning of this chapter. As you read through, consider where you are and where you would like to expand or make adjustments.

- What are your strengths?
- What areas do you wish to develop?

Learn

Consider the various practices that you learned about throughout this chapter.

- Which ones resonated most with you?
- Are there others not mentioned that you want to include in your self- or home-care routine?
- Which would you like to incorporate into your life?

- Are there any barriers that may hinder you?
- What resources do you need to support you?

Create a plan to guide you in incorporating these new practices and be-haviors. Consider including a timeline, adding in some things immediately, and layering in others over time.

Love

Over the next few weeks, begin building these practices into your regu-lar self- and home-care routine. Find creative ways to remind yourself and, where needed, simplify so the changes come more easily. Stay present and tuned into your body as you do each practice or make changes in your envi-ronment, noticing how you feel. Remain open and curious as you tune into and observe each layer—body, energy, mind, intellect, and spirit.

- What changes do you notice?
- Do you experience any difficulty or resistance with the practice?
- Are you experiencing the benefits you expected?

Continue to incorporate these practices and, over time, discern which prac-tices are providing the most benefit and where you may want to make adjust-ments.

Live

Once you have taken time to experiment and explore these practices, you will know which work best for your and your family's well-being and lifestyle. Continue to build on these throughout your daily life and make adjustments when needed. Remain mindful as you use these tools to bring the greatest benefit.

Chapter Summary

Technological advances have brought us tremendous benefits; however, they have also created challenges as we spend more and more time with our tech-nology and less time out in nature. In this chapter, we explored the conse-quences of these changes, as well as steps you can take to increase your con-nection with nature.

Paying attention to your environment and appreciating the natural world in the ways discussed in this chapter open new doors to ways to think about health. It means getting out into nature and bringing nature to you. And in our current world, it might mean taking steps to protect the natural world in any ways that feel appropriate and meaningful for you.

In the next chapter, we discuss how to create healthy attitudes toward finances.

nine

LETTING GO OF STRESS ABOUT MONEY

As covered in chapter 6 on transforming work stress, the path of karma yoga, also known as the yoga path of work, guides us to realize how our attachment to outcomes often results in disappointment and other stressful responses. We can apply this same principle to our relationship with money. Attachment to money, whether we consider ourselves wealthy or not, originates from familial and cultural beliefs we've internalized throughout our lives. Some of these beliefs create stress and anxiety about money and possessions, which negatively impacts our health on multiple levels. Money stress belongs to the person who is continually concerned with issues related to money. Someone earning a low income may not feel money stress depending on their situation or attitude. And on the other side, the millionaire fearful of losing his money or feeling pressed to earn one more million, is over focusing on money and experiencing stress.

In this chapter, we'll look at the many conflicted sources of our attitudes about money. You will have an opportunity to reflect on your own early money experiences and how they influenced you. Then we'll offer new perspectives that can guide you in altering your beliefs about money, alleviating stress in the process. The exercises and yoga practices will guide you to explore less stressful attitudes about finances and help you apply them in your life, to the benefit of your total health.

Familial and Cultural Messages About Money

As children, we received messages about money from varied sources. While many experts report that parents do not often talk to their children about money, experiences speak loudly and strongly. How much is or isn't available and how it is treated create the norms that we grow up to expect—or sometimes consciously reject—as adults. Parents' decisions about how to spend money and rules around working, chores, or allowance demonstrate values for children.

As children, we are also influenced by what we see around us in our communities. Who seems to have wealth and who doesn't? How are those people treated relative to one another? The impressions we formed may or may not be accurate, but they can have enormous influence on how we view, use, and relate to money.

Extreme conditions register strongly with children. The experience of not having enough to meet basic needs can be traumatic for a child (as well as adults). Good financial fortune can leave a positive or (perhaps unexpectedly) a negative imprint on children. As an example, Mom or Dad gets a raise and the family moves into a bigger house, and their daughter has to change schools. Depending on her response, she may learn to equate the increased money with exciting new changes, or with the loss of friends and familiarity.

Contradictory messages we receive about money in our larger culture through religion, politics, stories, and media also influence how we relate to money. Religions deliver explicit moral messages such as, "love of money is the root of all evil." Politicians debate the relative value of programs that, as they see it, either help the struggling poor, or cheat the hardworking and reward the lazy. Stories from *A Christmas Carol* to *The Simpsons* portray rich characters (Ebenezer Scrooge and Mr. Burns) as cheap, cold-hearted misers, and poor characters (like Cinderella and Charlie in *Charlie and the Chocolate Factory*) as virtuous and good. At the same time, reality TV and much of social media idolize the things that money can buy and the fabulously wealthy as people we should all emulate. Advertisements and images urge us to buy products in order to attain happiness. Our morals may give us one set of money guidelines and then our daily job may give us quite another. Small wonder if we feel confused!

Amid all these contradictory and confusing familial and cultural messages, each of us develops our own beliefs about what money is, what it means, and how we feel about it. We may not be consciously aware of what our beliefs are, but they drive many of our behaviors and choices. We can have upset stomachs or "worry ourselves sick" about money; we can ruin relationships by working overtime sixteen hours every day to reach our money goals. Rarely do people state that they are at peace with money, that they have enough, or that money is just a tool to us for the exchange of goods and services. The exercises and practices in this chapter will help illuminate how messages about finances influence your money mindset.

The Cost of Money Stress

Memories, attitudes, and beliefs about money along with fear of change and loss, combine to make finances the emotionally charged topic it is. And there's no doubt it is; about a quarter of American adults reported feeling extremely stressed about money. (Note that this figure was based on a survey conducted in 2015, a relatively stable year economically compared to the recession a few years earlier and widespread unemployment that would follow. We can imagine how much the data collected would differ in difficult times.)

If you have felt stressed about money recently, you're far from alone. In an annual survey conducted by the American Psychological Association, finances were reported as the top stressor for nine consecutive years.[32] The 2015 study, significantly titled "Paying With Our Health," reported 72 percent of adults felt stressed about money some of the time, and about one-quarter of adults reported that stress to be extreme.[33] People in the study with lower incomes reported higher levels of stress as did younger adults and parents. Also revealed was worry about money becoming a life-long pattern: Twenty-somethings worry

---

32. Starting in 2016, concerns related to political climate and the future of our country replaced money as the primary source of stress.

33. American Psychological Association, "Stress in America: Paying with Our Health," February 2015. https://www.apa.org/news/press/releases/stress/2014/stress-report.pdf.

about securing a job that will pay for the life they want to build; parents worry about saving for college and retirement; and seniors worry about living on a fixed income.

Worry about finances inevitably bleeds over into other health areas. We fear how our lives might change in the face of job loss or reduced income, dwelling on what-ifs that can keep us up at night. We compare our finances to others' and worry that we aren't keeping up, which affects our mental health. The quality of the food we eat and the nutrition it offers may be influenced by beliefs about what is appropriate to spend on food. Arguments about money are a leading cause of relationship stress, sometimes leading to divorce.[34]

Yet more money isn't the solution. Even billionaire investors worry about catastrophic investments or economic downturns if their beliefs about money are tied to a mindset of lack, a fear-based point of view where nothing is ever enough. So for the sake of your health, it's important to learn ways to adjust any unhealthy attitudes you might have that create stress about money. That process begins—as you might have guessed!—with identifying your underlying beliefs.

EXERCISE My Money Story Baseline

Understanding your own money story is the first step in understanding the beliefs that cause undue money stress and affect your health. Then with valuable insight in hand, you can begin to make changes that will be an asset to your total health.

Below are a series of questions to ask yourself about the origins of your views on money. Take your time to consider them and write down your answers in your journal. As you reflect on your money history, be as honest as you can with yourself. Honor the memories that stand out. If you remember a parent or businessperson using money in some pivotal manner, or delivering a message that resonated with you, explore that memory. Out of the hundreds of money-related interactions you experienced growing up, your

---

34. Lorraine Harvey, "As 'Divorce Day' Looms, Money Worries Top List of Reasons Why Married Couples Will Split in 2018," https://www.slatergordon.co.uk/media-centre /press-releases/2018/01/as-divorce-day-looms-money-worries-top-list-of-reasons-why -married-couples-will-split-in-2018/.

mind held on to that one, so chances are it shaped your viewpoint in a significant way. Also remember that there are no right or wrong answers, just your individual story. Even siblings who grew up in the same circumstances may respond differently.

Present-Day Associations

- What comes to mind when you think about money?
- What feelings do you experience when you think about money?
- What is your dominant emotion related to money?
- Do you believe in abundance (there is enough for everyone) or scarcity (resources are limited, there isn't enough to go around)?
- What do you believe about your current financial situation?
- What do you believe is the purpose of money?
- How do beliefs about money influence how you perceive others?

Past Associations

- How did your mother, father, and/or other guardian each talk about money?
- How did money effect your family of origin? Were there arguments, tension, or appreciation?
- How did you approach money as a child? Were you a saver? A spender? Or were you indifferent?
- What pivotal events in your childhood shaped your views related to money?

Insights Gained

Consider what you learned about yourself by answering these questions. Identify one view or belief about money that is negatively affecting your health. Write down the belief and all the ways you feel this view impacts you in unhealthy ways.

Next, take the insights that you have now into a situation that you experienced as a child. Visualize your adult self giving your younger self some ideas on how to handle the particular money-stress situation. This can help heal the emotional associations that similar present-day situations may evoke.

EXERCISE Transforming Your View of Wealth

To start transforming your view of money, take a moment and imagine seven piggy banks lined up in a row, labeled as follows:

- Emotional Fulfillment
- Finances
- Health
- Hobbies, Interests, and Enjoyable Activities
- Intellectual Fulfillment
- Relationships
- Spiritual Fulfillment

Imagine that each bank contains the wealth of experiences you've accumulated over your lifetime thus far. Write down or draw your unique experiences, values, and qualities that you would place in each one. See how much overall life-wealth you have accumulated in each area. It will probably be easier to start with positive experiences, successes. Then see if you can use "lessons learned" to find benefits from less than advantageous experiences.

Be creative as you mentally fill your piggy banks. For example, if your finance piggy bank is full, that's wonderful. However, how about you have little money at the moment but you have a clear plan for your retirement savings, one that relieves pressure because you know that in 20 years, your savings will grow. That's another way that your finance piggy bank can be full. What if your fitness routine is strong and you have learned to love exercise, so it is very easy? Consider fitness your hobby or interest. You may be a millionaire of fitness! Or, you are working hard and are busy, so your hobbies are suffering presently. You can easily remedy this by counting play time with your children as a hobby, and suddenly you're rich in your hobby piggy bank.

Let this exercise guide you toward small changes in your life. If your intellect seems dry, then start listening to something that stimulates your mind during your commute to work. Spiritually, you may need to assess how to manage that and recognize that simply adopting a compassionate attitude turns your work into a spiritual activity. The possibilities for bringing riches to each area of your life are endless!

Receiving Wealth in a Variety of Ways

It is one step to fill your piggy bank with various types of energy, to receive the energy is a second step. For some, the art of receiving is challenging. Past events, beliefs, and ways in which we are socialized affect how easy or difficult it is for individuals to feel worthy of receiving. This may be evident in various aspects, not just with money. For example, some people have difficulty receiving compliments, asking for or receiving help when needed or offered, or receiving love.

Our ability to receive help, gifts, compliments, money, love, or other things often reflects upon our sense of core worthiness. While some may lie on one end of the spectrum or the other—unable to receive or find it very easy to receive—most of us lie somewhere along the continuum. We receive certain things easily but struggle with others, or are able to receive but only to a limited extent. As an example, you receive enough income to cover the bills and necessities; however, you do not experience a sense of abundance of wealth flowing to you. The following exercises are designed to help you flex your receiving muscles and expand your ability to let abundance flow into your experience.

EXERCISE Expanding Receptivity

First, reflect on your level of receptivity using the following questions to guide you. Consider your thoughts, how your body feels, and any emotional response you experience in these situations. Write your insights in your journal to refer to later.

- When you need help with something, do you readily ask someone to assist you or do you avoid requesting help? Do you make a list of reasons why help is not accessible to you?

- If someone compliments you, how do you feel? Are you able to receive the compliment with ease? Do you deflect it by making a dismissive or diminishing statement, or a joke? Does it feel comfortable to receive or awkward?

- What do you do when someone offers to buy you dinner, pays for a cup of coffee, or gives you a gift? Are you able to accept graciously? Do you argue with them or try to reject their offering? What do you feel in your body in these moments?

163

- How do you handle money conversations with your employer, clients or contractors? For example, on a job interview, how do you handle the discussion about salary?

- Consider other experiences when you have had the opportunity to receive from others and note how you responded. Think of times when you were offered love, attention, support, and so forth.

Over the next few weeks, practice expanding your ability to receive. Start small if you need to, then as you start getting more comfortable, practice receiving things that are more challenging for you. Notice opportunities throughout your day. As people offer common courtesies such as holding a door for you or wishing you well, recognize that these are gifts that are being offered and allow yourself to receive them and feel appreciation. The next time someone offers to help you with something, accept their assistance. When complimented, pause, take a breath, and allow yourself to receive the compliment fully and without deflection. When you need help with something, practice asking for assistance. Understand that if receiving is challenging for you, this practice will feel a little uncomfortable at first. That is normal, but the discomfort will lessen as you strengthen your receiving muscles.

Reframing Your Money Mindset

In order to reframe your image or viewpoint on money, first contemplate the source of your views. For example, if George repeatedly denies himself material items using the statement "Money doesn't grow on trees," he can research the origins of this comment. Perhaps he remembers his grandmother saying this statement over and over when he was younger because his grandfather had expensive taste in cars and clothing. So, the essence of George's behavior is fear of being a spender like his grandfather, as he doesn't want to be rebuked by the echo of his grandmother's angry admonishment. As a result of his self-searching, George can set a new image that heals this situation by thinking of something that allows his identity to be measured by non-material items or by good acts instead of whether or not he buys expensive clothes. So, his slogan could be "George is a kind man." This may seem unrelated to money, but it changes the model of self-esteem based on appearance to self-esteem based on kindness.

EXERCISE Changing Your Money Statements

Look at your journal entries from the initial exercise in this chapter. What are the common themes and beliefs that you carry regarding money? Identify the internal and external messages that limit your sense of abundance.

On a clean page, draw a line down the center. In the left column, write down each of the limiting messages that you tell yourself about money. Following the above example, establish the underlying root of the message. Then in the right column, create new statements that free you from each of the limiting messages.

Yoga and Money

As members of a consumer culture, we tend to identify with the things we own. Social scientists refer to this as the "extended self," the idea that our belongings are a part of who we are.[35]

There's nothing wrong with buying things we like that will enrich our lives or make them easier. It is identifying with objects that can set us up for problems and stress. Spending on things we can't afford puts us into debt, compounding our stress. And while we all know better than that in theory, for some of us the urge is very difficult to resist. Some people meet their desire to buy by working harder or longer hours rather than going into debt, but this path includes its own pitfalls. Work itself is often stressful, and logging excessive time can strain relationships, as well as limit time for the health pillars of exercise, good nutrition, and sleep. Finally, hitching our identities to a constant stream of possessions creates spiritual stress, marked by persistent, nagging feelings of discontent, inadequacy, and of never having or being enough.

Yoga teachings offer an alternate view on possessions. According to the yoga concept known as *aparigraha* (translated as "non-greed"), identifying with our possessions creates an inner confusion. If we become attached to possessions, they become burdens that weigh us down and cloud our minds. When we care too much for our possessions, *they* control *us*, not the other way around. We find ourselves devoting our time and energy to obtaining

---

35. Russell W. Belk, "Possessions and the Extended Self," *Journal of Consumer Research* 15, 2: 139–168. September 1988. https://doi.org/10.1086/209154.

possessions, maintaining them, and safeguarding them from harm. In yoga, the people who see life clearly are the people who may own possessions but do not become attached to them. Their identities remain strong and independent with or without the things they might own. That person is unburdened by emotional reactions that come when an object is lost or damaged. There's a freedom that comes with not depending on external objects to feel complete.

The concept of ego suggests that we may buy things to show our value or worth. If we can afford a big house or an expensive car, maybe we believe it shows that we are capable, successful people. Purchasing can also show that we belong to a group. If everyone we socialize with always buys the newest, most advanced technology, we may want to keep up too. For some people, keeping up might mean spending a lot of money to be thin, or charitable, or "green." While most of us would consider the ends worthwhile, yoga places importance on the intent. It matters whether we are acting for the benefit of our health, the good of others, or to prove (to others or ourselves) that we can take that action.

EXERCISE Replacing Attachments with Ease

Examining the reasons behind our attachments to specific objects can shed light on our attachments, and perhaps help direct us to an alternate path toward fulfilling that need. List objects you feel attached to or objects you want badly but can't afford. Notice the response in your body when you visualize each one. Choose one you have the strongest response to and ask yourself these questions:

- What does the object represent to me?
- Is there another way I can fulfill that same need? For example, if you are drawn to something beautiful but too expensive, are there other ways for you to bring beauty into your home or your life? If it reminds you of a person or a time in your life that makes you happy, do you still need a physical representation of that memory?
- After reflecting, use breathing techniques, yoga poses, meditation, and other practices to help you create a healthy distance between your identity and your possessions, allowing yourself to hold them a bit

more lightly. For example, pause and observe your breath for a few moments. Notice the lungs open from low in the abdominal region, widening through the rib cage area, and finally lifting the upper chest. Now as you exhale, notice the tranquility as the air slowly leaves the lungs. As you do this, life slows down and you start to notice your internal state of mind. Your nervous system calms, and you feel a sense of relaxation. Your mood uplifts. All this occurred with no external aid, you can be simply content to be alive.

Use Resources

A last note: in chapter 7 we talked about avidya, or a spiritual sort of ignorance. Overcoming avidya is essential regarding money, as it is for all stress, but in this case we may need external, worldly knowledge as well. Money management is complicated, and most of us aren't sufficiently educated in how to do it, which in itself creates stress. Ask yourself honestly whether you need to learn more about money management, and if so, commit to that goal and give it a deadline. It's the kind of thing we often put off, but our health pays the price. Look into articles, books, podcasts, and other resources to raise your financial literacy. If you believe it is warranted, seek referrals for a professional to help you wade through financial information and how it applies to your unique situation. The Financial Therapy Association provides information and referrals for practices that take both financial information and emotional issues into account, for individual and couples.[36] Finally, consider consulting a yoga therapist for help in examining and transforming any embedded beliefs about money that may be permeating the way you look at the world and yourself.

EXERCISE Your Personalized Plan for Creating
Healthy Attitudes Toward Money

Earlier you read a series of questions about money in your life. We covered money in the past and the present. What about the future? Pause to envision a future without money stress, then ask yourself the following questions.

---

36. The Financial Therapy Association, https://www.financialtherapyassociation.org/.

- What would it mean to you to be free from stress about money?
- What beliefs would you have to modify?
- What other actions would you have to take?

Now that you have examined your personal money story and explored several practices to shift limiting patterns and beliefs about money, it is time to determine how to integrate what you have learned into your life. Develop a plan for improving your relationship with money and your attitude about it. Reflect on your experiences and review journal entries from this chapter. You have established your money story baseline and explored a variety of factors that may be limiting your ability to have a healthy relationship with money. Through these practices, you have discovered your strengths as well as your limitations surrounding money. Consider these questions:

- What are my financial strengths? Challenges?
- What would I most like to see change in my financial situation?
- What would it mean to be free from stress about money? How would my life change?
- What beliefs do I need to modify that are limiting my ability to receive money abundantly?
- What behaviors are hindering me?
  - What steps do I need to take to shift those behaviors?
- What resources are available to help support my goals?
- What action steps are needed?
- What will I see as evidence that I am successful in achieving my goals?

Using the SMART format that you learned in chapter 3, write out your goals in your journal. Identify the *specific goal(s)* that you wish to achieve, when and how. Determine how you will *measure* your success, both short term and overall. Establish what you need to *attain* your goal, including internal and external resources. Write out why this is *relevant* and important to you—get clear on your motivations. Lastly, establish a reasonable *timeline* for reaching your goal.

Chapter Summary

Money stress exists at all phases of life and for people of all tax brackets. Knowing your belief system related to money can help free you from patterns that create stress. You can revise your money beliefs as a means of living fully, rich or poor. Planning for your future is a way to minimize worry and live fully.

This chapter concludes our section on social health. The lifestyle areas of work, relationships, environment, and money each play a separate and interconnected role in our total health. The next section is on intrapersonal health, namely, recreation, meditation, and spirituality. These three areas complete our journey through each area of life, allowing us to empower our health from every angle. Small adjustments in each of the lifestyle areas lead to major improvements in health.

part four
INTRAPERSONAL HEALTH

This section on intrapersonal health will help you examine your beliefs about spirituality and devise a plan to nourish your spirit that, in turn, uplifts your health. Chapter 10 invites you to appreciate the healthful effects of joy and recreation in your life. Chapter 11 offers guidelines for how to develop a personal meditation practice. Chapter 12 helps you tap into your spirituality and connect it to your healthy lifestyle.

Ten

MAKING TIME FOR JOY AND RECREATION

With everything we need to be responsible for in our lives—finances, work, relationships, and our environment—plus taking care of ourselves through sleep, nourishment, and fitness, it's only natural to ask: When is there time for enjoyment? When do I get to do my hobbies, play, laugh, and have some good old fun? The Comprehensive Yoga therapy answer to that question goes something like this: When you value those things as essential to your health and make time for them.

The yogic path of the intellect is a helpful guide when it comes to recognizing the value of joy and recreation in our lives. This path is more than simply about knowledge or knowing, rather it's about *direct experience*—a real-time, tangible, embodied experience where we are connected to the present moment and aware of how we are feeling. From that awareness, we come to understand how specific people, places, and things contribute positively or negatively to our well-being. We can then incorporate that information into our choices about how, when, and with whom we spend our time and energy. This chapter explores why joy and recreation are vital parts of our comprehensive health. The exercises and yoga practices will get you thinking about your beliefs about and attitudes toward joy and recreation. They'll provide opportunities to craft a plan that integrates hobbies and other uplifting activities into your life.

The Health Benefits of Creative Hobbies

One of the biggest regrets expressed by hospice patients at the end of their lives is, "I wish that I had let myself be happier."[37] Although each of us defines happiness differently, what is most important is that we purposefully carve out time to do the things that contribute to our happiness. For full health, it's necessary to approach joy and recreation with the same enthusiasm that you bring to physical health, work, finances, and the other lifestyle areas discussed in this book. Activities that lift our mood, bring ease into our body and mind, or spark creativity nourish our being in ways that no amount of healthy nutrition or financial success can.

We shortchange ourselves when we view leisure only as an "escape" from responsibilities, yet that is what many of us do. According to theorists, the escape mentality leads to spending our free time primarily in passive pursuits such as watching television. And while there may be a positive place for TV in our lives (more on this soon), it can become a habit to only watch TV or be on our devices during downtime. Passive activities can lead to boredom, which can turn to apathy and eventually depression. Creative hobbies, on the other hand, provide opportunities to enrich and re-energize ourselves in a proactive way.[38] There are even studies that show people who engage in creative hobbies feel more relaxed, have a better sense of mastery and control, and are more creative and helpful at work.

Many activities can qualify as a creative hobbies, including needlework, gardening, woodwork, sports, painting, creative writing, playing a musical instrument, and so many others, but it depends on how you approach them. The point of a creative hobby is its personal nature. That is, hobbies provide

---

37. Bronnie Ware, "The Regrets of the Dying," https://bronnieware.com/blog/regrets-of-the-dying/.

38. Fred R.H. Zijlstra, Sabine Sonnentag, "After Work Is Done: Psychological Perspectives on Recovery from Work," *European Journal of Work and Organizational Psychology* 15 (2): 129–138. June 2006. DOI: 10.1080/13594320500513855.

opportunities for personal growth and offer a sense of challenging yourself, giving you a chance to develop new thought processes and skills.[39] A hobby is also something you choose to do out of your own interest, not out of need or assignment. And there is nothing riding on your results. You can think of it this way: Cooking for pay in a restaurant is work. Cooking the same set of dishes every week is an efficient way to feed a family. Finding new recipes to try, experimenting with new ingredients and techniques, taking risks and sometimes failing, transforms cooking into a hobby.

For example, in her youth Carol wanted to be a doctor like her mother, who was a pioneer in woman's health care. However, Carol's high aptitude for writing caused her teachers and parents to encourage her to pursue writing as a career, although it was not her passion. Eventually, Carol completed her PhD in English and had a rewarding teaching career. After reflecting in yoga therapy sessions as to why she loved yoga so much, she saw that it rekindled her love of health and healing that she had unknowingly suppressed. While nearing retirement, Carol decided to train more fully in yoga as a healing modality as well as in herbalism. Eventually, Carol linked her writing to healthy living and merged her talents with her passion.

EXERCISE List Your Hobbies

In your journal, take some time to name hobbies that you have enjoyed throughout your life.

- What did you enjoy as a child?
- What hobbies did you give up as a kid and why?
- How do your hobbies reflect your personality?
- Do you still enjoy any of these hobbies, and if so, how often do you engage in them?
- Are there creative ways that you can weave hobbies into your present life?

---

39. Council for Disability Awareness, "How Hobbies are Healthy." http://blog.disability canhappen.org/hobbies-are-healthy/.

The Joy of Play

Children's play is easy to recognize, but it's harder to describe in adults. In 2017, the *International Journal of Play* dedicated a special issue to adult play, drawing attention to it as an understudied area within psychology. Yet as far back as 1938, psychology researchers referred to a need for adults to "relax, amuse oneself, seek diversion and entertainment; have fun, play games, laugh, joke, and be merry."[40] Like hobbies, play is something you do because you want to, but unlike knitting or gardening, usually there is no product involved. Play is done completely for its own sake.

Given our busy and goal-oriented lives, play doesn't register with many adults. We have too many other things to do. Playing might feel irresponsible, childish. If this is true for you, think about where that attitude comes from. Is there a hidden belief behind it? Is it one you'd like to change? There are good reasons to do so. Experts call play uniquely and intrinsically rewarding. It generates optimism, seeks out novelty, makes perseverance fun, leads to mastery, gives the immune system a little boost, fosters empathy, and promotes a sense of belonging and community."[41]

EXERCISE The Feeling of Play

Tap into your sense of play by thinking back to your much younger self. Ask yourself:

- What did you like to do as a child?
- Did you like to play pretend? Build things? Draw?
- How did those activities make you feel?
- Did you lose track of time while doing your favorite activity?
- Can those memories inspire you to reclaim an old activity?

Of course, being an adult is different from being a child, and the ways you play now will look and feel different, but play can still bring joy as an adult. It

---

40. Henry A. Murray, "Explorations in Personality: A Clinical and Experimental Study of Fifty Men of College Age," Originally published 1938, Oxford University Press.

41. Rene T. Proyer, ""A Multidisciplinary Perspective on Adult Play and Playfulness," *Journal of Play* 6 (3): 241. 2017. https://www.tandfonline.com/doi/full/10.1080/21594937.2017 .1384307.

depends on how you approach it. Teaching a favorite activity or board game to your child is its own kind of joy. Hanging with adult friends at a backyard barbecue can serve the same purpose as giggling with childhood playmates, if you truly allow yourself to relax and have a good time. Playing a sport like tennis or basketball can be a joyful form of fitness when approached with a light heart.

If you need a jump-start, you can search online for the toys you used to play with as a child, or better yet, find a toy store, art- or school-supply store and walk down the aisles. Skip over the electronic toys that respond to the push of the button. Instead, look for items that require you to use your hands and your imagination. Following is a list of old favorites that might serve as a spark.

- Googly eyes
- Silly putty
- Crayons
- Frisbees
- Bubbles with a wand to blow
- Modeling clay or play dough
- Board games
- Magnifying glass (use it to scope bugs outside)
- Tennis ball
- Playground ball
- Beach ball
- Sled
- Hula hoop
- Deck of cards
- Bubble wrap!

Also keep in mind that a playful spirit can arise in other activities, even boring ones. Young children seem to play endlessly with bubbles. Can you recall a bit of that sense of wonder just for a moment, as you do the dishes?

And why not toss the balled socks into the laundry basket as if you're shooting baskets?

The Power of Joyful Thinking

Stress gets in the way of joy. Sometimes the stress comes from being too busy or worried or both. Much of this book is about learning to let go of stress. Establishing balanced habits that promote physical health and good sleep improves our ability to address stressful situations. Learning new approaches to work, relationships, our environment, and finances transforms habits and beliefs that add to stress. But stress still happens, and sometimes it's almost like stress becomes a habit.

In fact, stress can become a habit. Back in chapter 1 we covered the way in which performing the same actions or repeating the same thoughts carves a path within the neurons in our brains, almost like shoveling a path through snow. The more we use the path, the wider and clearer it gets, and the more automatically our brains will follow it. When we spend a lot of time stressing, worrying about "what if?" and "oh, no, but...", that worry pathway becomes our brain's go-to pattern.

The good news is that we can change our brain habits with purposeful, joyful thinking. By developing different habits of thought, we can shovel new pathways. The old ones won't disappear, but they can become old and worn when replaced by new, clearer, wider pathways. Distraction can be a useful technique. If you notice yourself engaging in fruitless worry or caught in a spiral of thinking that is getting you nowhere, stop and do something else that is more neutral in nature or connects you to joy. Yoga poses, breathing, exercising, petting an animal, calling a friend, or starting a task can all interrupt your thought pattern and give yourself something else to do. Like any new habit, this will take practice, so keep your expectations in check at first, then watch as it becomes easier.

Let's focus on how yoga poses can help. At the same time you are engaging your body in movement, you can teach your brain to follow new patterns of thought by connecting the movement with uplifting mantras or affirmations. If you attend a yoga class or try some movement-based activity, notice how it makes you feel. Try approaching movement the way you would approach a hobby: Lift your arms up and smile; lean forward and sigh. Take some time for relaxation. Swing your body like a rag doll and see what you notice.

As you find different areas of your life where you can insert a joyful attitude, you will reprogram your mind to recognize that joy can be found in traffic, at work, and at deadline time. While we usually choose to find stress in situations we deem unpleasant, it is also possible to find positives by having a childlike, joyful attitude. This change in attitude does great things for your body, mind, and spirit!

The Bright Side Game

In a technique called the Bright Side game, you can match each of your negative thoughts with a new, positive one. It would go something like this, "I didn't have time to get to the grocery store and we're low on food." Now instead of panicking or beating yourself up for not being organized, think of something positive: "But on the bright side, now I have a reason to finish up those leftovers, and I'll save money besides." Or "I'm so busy at work this week! But on the bright side, all that work will keep me from worrying too much about the meeting with my son's teacher."

Feel free to use humor in your bright side thinking to more fully lighten the load. "I can't believe I caught a cold! The holidays are coming and I don't have time for this! But on the bright side, I could really use a day to catch up at home. Plus it gives my nose a lovely Rudolph-esque glow!"

Gratitude

A lovely way to occupy your mind is to focus on gratitude. Numerous researchers have found an association between a sense of well-being and gratitude, defined as an appreciation of what is valuable and meaningful to you, or a general sense of thankfulness or appreciation. By consciously engaging in certain activities, you can foster a sense of gratitude and the associated well-being. Activities that may work include journaling about things you are grateful for, meditating on gratitude, practicing saying "thank you" in a sincere and meaningful way, and, if you are religious, praying about your gratitude.[42]

Gratitude doesn't have to be about the exciting or unexpected things that happen to you. When learning about this positive thinking exercise, most of us first think about big things, such as when your co-worker brought in lunch unexpectedly or your child tied their shoes for the first time. But if you had just been in a life-or-death experience, you would see things very differently. You would write down that you just took another breath. You saw your co-worker and it brought you joy. The little things start to count if you recognize that everything has a purpose and can be viewed as positive.

The Gratitude Game

Write down as many positive things as you can think of that happened to you today. To make it fun, set the clock for three minutes and go! Look at each item on your list. Take a moment to feel gratitude for each one. You can direct your gratitude at another person involved or just the fact that this happened. Repeat this exercise daily, weekly, or whatever period works for you. Over time, you can reach the final stage of this exercise, which is to realize that there is really no negative and positive, that simple existence can be valued. Thus, every thought you have can be counted in this exercise.

Protecting Your Joy

Besides adding to your new, more positive, thinking path, it's helpful to avoid walking in the old one. Be on your guard around negative people who draw you into their negative thinking. The goal isn't to avoid them, which is not a fully healthy response and may not be possible. But you can establish boundaries. If a friend calls you to vent too long or too often, try "I'm so sorry you feel that way. We talked about this problem yesterday and I really just don't have more to add. Is there something else you can do now to make yourself feel better?"

Also pay attention to the kind of messages you choose to receive A steady diet of sad books, crime dramas, horror movies, contentious political pro-

---

42. "Personal Health and Wellbeing" The National Institute for Play http://www.nifplay.org /opportunities/personal-health/.

gramming, and even the daily news all subject you to a tsunami of negativity. Stick to nourishing influences to maintain a healthy state of mind. (This relates back to the idea explored in chapter 4, that nourishment means not only the food you take into your body but also energies, emotions, and ideas.) If you feel a need to keep up with news, limit the time you spend and choose outlets that don't play to your emotions—namely fear, disgust, and anger.

Laughter Is the Best Medicine

Here's a joke: Why couldn't the yogi vacuum her apartment? Because she got rid of all her attachments![43]

Have you ever thought about what happens when you laugh? Most of us don't, but we're going to take laughter seriously for a just a moment because it can do seriously good things for your health.

Laughter is a full-brain, full-body, socially enhancing activity. In the brain, your frontal lobe, the limbic system (which regulates emotion), and motor cortex are all involved in hearing the joke or situation, deciding it's funny, and causing your body to respond. Your facial muscles contract. Your usual breathing pattern is disrupted as extra air is forced first out of and then into your lungs, boosting oxygen levels.[44] Your heart rate and blood pressure increase. Your core muscles contract and other muscles not used in laughter become temporarily weaker and less coordinated (as in the expression "fall down laughing").[45] And in your brain, your stress levels decrease and your immune system gets a boost.[46] Even just *anticipating* a good belly laugh pro-

43. "Yoga Jokes," Jokes4Us. http://www.jokes4us.com/sportsjokes/yogajokes.html.

44. Lindsay Wilson-Barlow, "The Psychological Effects of Laughter," findapsychologist.org, https://www.findapsychologist.org/the-physiological-effects-of-laughter-by-lindsay-wilson-barlow/.

45. SourceFed channel. "Science of Laughter," https://www.youtube.com/watch?v=OvfjYLU5ZXg.

46. Lee S. Berk, David L. Felten, Stanley A. Tan, Barry B. Bittman, James Westengard, "Modulation of neuroimmune parameters during the eustress of humor-associated mirthful laughter," *Alternative Therapies in Health and Medicine* 7(2): 62–72, 74–76. March 2001. https://www.ncbi.nlm.nih.gov/pubmed/11253418.

duces these healthy effects. And laughter helps people bond, making and strengthening social connections.[47]

Laughter even helps to heal trauma. A powerful story of laughter's healing power appears in the book *Calm Clarity* by social entrepreneur Due Quach (pronounced Zway Kwok). Due was born in Vietnam during the war to a family seeking to flee its terrible hardships. They succeeded when she was an infant, bringing her along on dangerous, frightening journeys to refugee camps and finally to America, where they were settled into what turned out to be a violent, gang-ridden part of Philadelphia. Her family struggled and opened a small take-out restaurant, where Due started working at the age of eight. Her family reached a state of stability, but poverty and violence remained in the backdrop of their lives.

Meanwhile, Due was an avid learner. She attended a top Philadelphia magnet high school and to her astonishment, was accepted to Harvard University. When she first got to Harvard, she writes "*... it was like walking on air.*"[48] The intellectual, affluent atmosphere felt like a dream. But over the course of her first eighteen months there, the dream collapsed. She felt both guilty for leaving her family behind and completely isolated in a sea of wealthy, privileged classmates. Her emotions triggered earlier traumatizing experiences of fear, insecurity, and discrimination, including experiences as an infant that she couldn't remember. When Due began experiencing panic attacks, including one that lasted for hours no matter what she did, she took herself to the emergency room.

Subsequent medication and therapy helped her get back on her feet, but she wanted more. Due decided to gain control over her life by learning everything she possibly could about neuroscience and then apply her knowledge to her own brain. From her studies, she determined that her early traumatic experiences had strengthened the neurocircuits in her mind that underlie negative emotion, meaning the way she felt was how she was predisposed to feel. She assigned herself the task of building up the brain circuits related to positive emotion instead. In *Calm Clarity*, Due writes, "By far the most effec-

---

47. BrainStuff – How Stuff Works, "How Does Laughter Work?" https://www.youtube.com /watch?v=FnZnbN3mQJ4.

48. Due Quach, *Calm Clarity: How to Use Science to Rewire Your Brain for Greater Wisdom, Fulfillment, and Joy* (New York: TarcherPerigree, 2018), 96.

tive mind-hacking idea I came up with was to laugh more. I started spending time every day watching comedy shows or movies that made me laugh hysterically. It worked... Instead of beating myself up whenever I experienced a setback, I created a habit of finding something funny in the situation or my own behavior to laugh at."[49]

Due graduated Harvard and went on to a successful business career. She founded a social enterprise company dedicated to empowering people of all backgrounds to, as she did, "overcome adversity and develop a mindset for growth, leadership, and resilience."[50]

Laughter Yoga

Relying on comedy for your laughter quotient is not a sure thing, however. You never know in advance if you'll find something funny enough for a good laugh. To ensure you get the physiological benefits, one answer is to simply laugh whether or not something is funny. This is where laughter yoga comes in. Normally, the laughter response begins when the right hemisphere of the brain decides something is funny. In laughter yoga, the response starts with the breath. There are many resources online for laughter yoga classes and clubs, so it is easy to find information of you'd like to join, or you can do it on your own. How? All you do is pretend to laugh until you start laughing for real. Begin by forcing air out of your lungs and saying "ha" repeatedly (or "hee," or "ho," whatever you like), in a pattern that imitates laughter. Stop, inhale, and repeat: HA HA ha ha ha ha ha! You can vary the pattern. HA ha ha ha HA ha ha HA ha ha. Or the syllables. HEE HEE ho ho ho ho ho!

After a short time of pretend laughter, the right hemisphere often joins in, deciding that sitting there saying "hee hee, ha, ha, ho, ho" about nothing is actually pretty funny. Then the forced laughter becomes as genuine as the health benefits it provides. This works especially well in a group, because laughter is contagious. What's more, the medical world is beginning to take seriously the therapeutic benefits of laughter, as the results of one study

---

49. Quach, *Calm Clarity*, 115..

50. Ibid., 25.

showed that laughter yoga subjects showed improvements in their mood after participating.[51]

EXERCISE Your Personalized Plan for Making
Time for Joy and Recreation

Set up a fun time plan. It might sound like an oxymoron to schedule in time to accomplish nothing productive in order to keep your mood light in all areas of your life. But trust us, fun is an essential component of overall health.

- List what is reasonable to expect in your present life.

- Transform activities into fun activities. Turn the need to cook into a hobby by experimenting. Or, turn babysitting into a time where you relearn to be a kid.

- Check your belief system to see if you think that joy can coexist with being a productive person. One of the most interesting observations of many people considered to be "great" people or "holy" leaders like the Dalai Lama is that these people smile, laugh, and then drop the most profound truths simultaneously.

- See how your smile becomes infectious within your body and with those around you.

Chapter Summary

Joyful thinking is like a vitamin for the soul. Laughter is a full-body experience and positively affects the systems of the body. Joking aside, laughter is in fact some of the best medicine out there! Please laugh a lot and often, and rekindle a love of hobbies, reintroducing them to your life. See the positive in situations by flipping negative statements into positive ones. Increase gratitude for the small things in life.

Now that you have learned about the health benefits of joy and recreation, let's move on to the role of meditation and relaxation as practices that

51. Rima Dolgoff-Kaspar, Ann Baldwin, M. Scott Johnson, Nancy Edling, Gulshan K. Sethi, "Effect of Laughter Yoga on Mood and Heart Rate Variability in Patients Awaiting Organ Transplantation: A Pilot Study," *Alternative Therapies in Health and Medicine* 18 (5): 61–66. Sep-Oct 2012.

also support your health. The meditation chapter is intentionally positioned after this one, on joy and recreation, so that you will carry a light and easy attitude into the discussion of meditation. It's often that meditation is seen as a difficult, serious task devoid of feeling. But as you'll see, meditation works best with a smile.

eleven

DEVELOPING A
MEDITATION PRACTICE

Although meditation has existed for centuries, it's trending now largely because of the changes in our high-tech world. To understand how, try this thought experiment: Take a few deep breaths and imagine it's two hundred years ago. Like most people of that time period, you live on a farm. You spend your days among plants and animals, doing hard, physical work. Most of the food you eat is from your own land. In the evening after supper, you sit and chat, perhaps do some sewing. And when the sun is down and the candles are low, you go to bed. The sounds you hear are all from nature, the only lights from the moon and the stars. There is no electricity, no blue or red glowing dots. Nothing beeps at all. Spend a few breaths in that scene, then look around at your present reality. Compare the two.

Whether the image of life long ago strikes you as idyllic or awful, it certainly feels very different from our current lives. Our human nervous systems were designed to live within that slow, steady, nature-centered pace. It's certainly true that the human system is adaptable; to an extent, humanity has been able to adjust to the constant stimulation built into modern living, but we have not adapted completely. Without natural lulls in our days, the mind can get overloaded. Our nervous systems spend a great deal less time in the calm "rest and digest" state, and a great deal more time feeling stressed and threatened.

The differences between the lifestyles of then and now account for meditation's current popularity. Two hundred years ago (and in fact until recent decades), meditation was primarily a spiritual or religious experience reserved for people interested in reaching deeper levels of consciousness. Now it draws many people who simply need to feel a sense of tranquility and rest.

As part of the raja path of yoga, related to knowing oneself, meditation and similar relaxation exercises are lifestyle habits whose goal is to deepen our self-understanding and bring clarity to our thought processes. Clarity leads to reduced stress and healthier life choices. In this chapter, you will learn a variety of relaxation exercises and six different styles of meditation from which you can choose the type(s) that most resonate with you. The last section of the chapter covers obstacles—things that tend to derail efforts to regularly meditate—and ways to manage or overcome them. Our goal is to give you all of the information you need so that when you're ready, you can establish and sustain your own meditation practice.

What Is Meditation?

Meditation is an activity done for the purpose of allowing the mind to calm. Humans have practiced it for thousands of years and still practice it around the world. Meditation is a central pillar of Eastern religions, including Taoism, Hinduism, and Buddhism. Judaism, Christianity, and Islam all include at least one branch in which meditation is practiced. Meditation (sometimes called trance awareness) is a foundation for all neo-Shamanistic or nature-based religions of the world. Even great scientists rely on deep, quiet thought in the process of discovery, a practice that is akin to meditation.

True meditation requires sitting quietly, usually for a minimum of twenty minutes, and turning the attention inward. Many activities that we think of as meditation, such as quiet periods listening to music or to someone speaking in a soothing tone, are considered relaxation or meditative activities, but not true meditation. This is because they draw our focus to something external to ourselves. They are still very valuable, however! In fact, most people fare better engaging in these kinds of activities before embarking on a true meditation practice. Meditation takes time and dedication. You can think of it as similar to long-distance running. If you're new to it, it's a poor idea to attempt a marathon your first day. But it's a great idea to start conditioning yourself, setting new goals that make sense for you over time.

There are a lot of claims out there about meditation. Some celebrities swear by it, and many influential businesspeople attribute their success to it. Individuals respond differently to meditation, so the claims made about it may or may not be true for you. But what is certain about meditation is that in the long run, it will bring you peace, and peace benefits health.

The same recent technological advances that enable us to learn about sleep also now allow Western scientific researchers to view the brain activity of advanced practitioners as they meditate. The resulting studies confirmsthat meditation reduces stress and also both strengthens and calms the mind. That feat may seem paradoxical if you haven't yet developed a meditation practice, but in time you will come to experience its truth. In short, research proves beyond a doubt that the meditation masters were right all along.

Preparing for Meditation with Relaxation

Settling the energy in your body—more specifically your nervous system— helps to prepare your mind to slow down in meditation. If you are new to meditation, we recommend integrating relaxation practices into your routine first. That way, you'll get used to slowing down as well as gain self-understanding about your reactions and responses to these kinds of activities.

To gain the benefits of relaxation, set aside a few minutes each day in a quiet place to come into a resting state. Before bed often works, and so do other times of the day, depending on what feels best to you and the activity you are doing. As you recall from the chapter on sleep, brains are in a restful state when brain waves reach the alpha level, a kind of quasi-sleep. Here are some suggestions for relaxation activities you can integrate right away into your comprehensive health routine.

Gentle Movement

A good practice is to bend the spine in five directions. You can do this standing freely, standing and holding onto a chair for support, or seated.

1. First, stretch upward toward the sky. Keeping your spine long, bend toward the right, back to the middle, and then the left, stretching the muscles along the sides of your body.

2. Next, allow your head, neck, and shoulders to roll forward until you are reaching down toward the floor.

3. Then reverse the movement, rolling upward and raising your arms up overhead again or holding on to the chair, and bend slightly backwards.

4. Finally, reach your right arm toward your left thigh and then vice versa, for a gentle twist.

While you are moving, practice deep breathing and a mindset of letting go. Make an active decision to not think about your to-do list or whatever is worrying or annoying you today. Concentrate instead on the here and now. If you notice other thoughts return, that's okay. Simply refocus.

Now choose one or more of the following relaxation exercises.

Body Scan

For this relaxation, you are welcome to sit or lie comfortably.

1. Mentally scan your body from the crown of your head to the soles of your feet, moving slowly and purposefully through all the parts of your body and differentiating between left and right sides.

2. As you do, you may notice areas where you are holding on to tension. As you notice tension, exhale to try to let it release.

3. Continue your scan. When you reach your feet, if you aren't too sleepy, you can do it again, this time perhaps toes to crown.

4. See if you can allow the tense areas to relax a little more.

Sixteen Points

This ancient practice is related to the body scan but guides your awareness to sixteen specific points along your body. Perform this relaxation on your back.

As you breathe, notice the following points in order. Take at least one long, slow breath on each point.

1. Tips of the toes
2. Ankles
3. Knees
4. Fingertips
5. Tailbone
6. Lower belly (Note your breathing!)
7. Navel
8. Belly, between navel and ribcage
9. Heart
10. Throat (Release your neck and shoulders.)
11. Lips (Release your jaw.)
12. Tip of the nose
13. Eyes
14. Space between your eyebrows (Also called the third eye.)
15. Forehead (Let this remind you again to release any worry.)
16. Crown of the head

If you fall asleep during this exercise, that's okay. It's a sign you are a bit sleep deprived, and it's great that this relaxed you into sleep. In fact, you might want to do it in bed regularly to encourage sleep. But if you don't want to fall asleep, try doing it a little earlier in the evening or day.

Emphasis on the Exhale

For this relaxation exercise, lie on the floor on your belly instead of your back.

1. Let your arms be a pillow beneath your forehead, chin, or cheek. (To avoid strain on your neck, be sure to alternate sides if you lie on your cheek.)
2. Hinge your right hip out toward the right wall and bend your right knee, so the inner part of your thigh and calf is resting on the floor.

3. Drag your right thigh upward along the floor a little so your hip is at more or less a 45-degree angle, with your inner thigh and calf still resting on the ground. The point of this is to get very comfortable. If you aren't, adjust your positioning until you are.

4. Breathe in this relaxed position, especially noticing the exhale, which will be longer than the inhale and might include a small sigh.

5. The weight on your belly promotes that feeling of a sigh as you exhale. Take advantage of the feeling to continue releasing any tension as you sigh.

Square Breathing

This breathing exercise is a helpful technique for taking slow, long breaths.

1. To begin, breathe slowly and count the number of seconds it takes for you to inhale, and then to exhale. Most beginners count about three seconds, more experienced yogis will count higher. See if you can extend your inhale and your exhale to one second longer than your natural count was, so if your count for both was five, try to extend to six. Also try to make them even, so if your first count was four-inhale and three-exhale, first make them both four. Then see if you can extend both to five or six. Now continue breathing to the longer, even count.

2. Next, bring your attention to the small pause that happens between the inhale and the exhale. Normally, that is less than one second. But you are going to lengthen that, as well. Staying with the example of four: Inhale for a count of four. Then gently hold the breath inside your lungs for four.

3. Now exhale for four seconds, then "hold" the exhale for four.

4. Continue in this even breathing pattern for several rounds, staying calm and relaxed as you do. Repeat if you like.

Relax and Visualize

This exercise works well for people who are very visual or have strong imaginations. It can be done in any comfortable position.

1. Sit or lie quietly and begin breathing.

2. Imagine a scene that you find soothing. It might be the beach, a meadow, a mountaintop, a room in front of a cozy fire. Place yourself in the scene.

3. Scan the scene in your mind, seeing all the different sights there are to view.

4. Hear its sounds. Sniff its odors. Continue this relaxation exercise for up to ten minutes.

A variation to practice if your daily worries persist as you visualize is this: Imagine a basket in the scene. When an unwelcome thought comes up, imagine that you are placing that thought in the basket. Remind yourself that it will wait for your attention another time.

Meditation for Your Lifestyle

Years ago as part of his dissertation thesis, your author Bob Butera outlined six major types of meditation based on the multiple meditation traditions from around the world, both East and West. The six types include: breath; visualization and affirmation; mantra; prayer, devotion, or intentionality; contemplative inquiry; and mindfulness. None of these types is better than another, but different ones sit better with different people. There doesn't seem to be any formula to calculate in advance which form of meditation will work best for you, but you can observe your responses to the different types to help you choose. The best thing is to go with what appeals to you and see how it works. You might have to try a few types before settling on one that feels right.

EXERCISE Observe Your Natural Meditation Method

Take five minutes and sit quietly. That's it—sit quietly. The how, when, and where is entirely up to you.

The purpose of this exercise is to observe your natural inclinations when you are quiet. Make a note in your journal about your experience and what you did during the quiet time. Note any sort of mental distractions you had or the types of thoughts or feelings you experienced, as well as what you did during the quieter, peaceful moments. You will do part 2 of this exercise after reading about the various types of meditation.

Types of Meditation

1. Breathing

You learned in the chapter on movement and in the relaxation exercises earlier in this chapter that conscious breathing is a good way to calm the nervous system, making you feel more relaxed and calmer. Meditation that highlights the breath takes this fact to another level. Many meditation practices use breath as a supporting or secondary technique, but in this tradition it is primary.

The mind, as you know, is drawn to things in the material world that attract its attention—a car horn, a harsh light, someone walking into the room. With attention scattered outward in that way, the mind is unable to turn inward. A smooth, steady, even breath is the doorway that allows the mind to step inside. Breathing this way sharpens the mind so that it can center in on one place, like a spotlight. A focused mind can illuminate deeper parts within yourself, allowing them to be seen and understood.

When the breath is uneven, the mind's energy becomes diffuse again and the attention returns to the outside world. If you've never observed your breath, you might be surprised at how often it is choppy, or erratic, or comes in gasps. Learning how to make it smooth and even is a first step in this style of meditation. There are varying techniques for doing this. One is to sit quietly and focus your awareness on the air moving in and out of the throat (the bronchial tubes). That's it—just sit, focus, and breathe.

This practice is simple and profound but can be difficult to sustain for a length of time, as the mind becomes easily distracted. Including a spiritual element offers something to more easily occupy the mind, as well as enriches the experience. You can think about inhaling the qualities you want to imbue yourself with, such as gratitude or love. You can breathe out negative qualities you need to rid yourself of, such as fear or anger. Or you can both inhale and exhale positive qualities you want to gain from and share with the world. Let your mind ponder the words as you breathe. Breathing equals life itself, so there is much to contemplate.

Or you can keep your concentration on your own body. In yoga, breath is energy. When you inhale and exhale, energy fills your lungs and flows around inside you. For example, you can breathe into your belly, or your feet, or your third eye, the spot a little ways above the space between your eyebrows. During breathing meditation, a focus on breathing into the different parts of your body can stimulate different types of energy.

An especially uplifting version of the breathing meditation adds a smile to the action. Called the Inner Smile meditation in the Taoist tradition, in this style you sit and breath with a small smile on the lips. As you breathe, when thoughts or other distraction arise, simply greet them with a smile. It doesn't take long for the lifted facial muscles to translate into a lifted mood as well!

2. Visualization and Affirmation

Visualizations are a concentrated form of the very common activity of imagining something in your mind. When paired with affirmations—positive, declarative statements—they help us let go of our everyday selves and understand that there is more to the world than we humans can see from our limited perspectives. This type of meditation consists of repeating the affirmation while contemplating the visual image.

The affirmations we are talking about here can be tied to practical goals or concerns that are essentially spiritual in nature (so an affirmation such as "I will win the lottery" doesn't qualify but affirmations related to values such as appreciating health do). Visualizations add another dimension to the affirmations and make them easier to believe in. The goal is to reach deeper levels of the unconscious where true and lasting change can occur. (More on using spirituality to accomplish practical goals appears in the next chapter).

Simply repeating a phrase you hear somewhere or that someone else tells you is effective but not enough to make an affirmation. The phrase has to resonate with you personally. You may need to try out several and be creative to discover one that works.

Because affirmation and visualization are effective together at reaching into our subconscious, it's common for unbidden thoughts, images, and observations to arise. The goal is to notice what comes up, refocus on the meditation, and come back to the subconscious thought later, trying to deduce what it means. Often it involves beliefs we were taught or picked up as children. Now as adults, we can look at them and decide to hold on to them or work to let them go.

3. Mantra

A mantra is the repetition of a phrase, word, or syllable for the duration of the meditation practice. The power of the mantra comes from the internal vibration created by the word combined with its meaning. In some traditions, including Transcendental Meditation, the mantra is given from teacher to student in a ceremony. In other practices, people simply choose their own. Often the mantra comes from religious teaching, such as a short phrase or single word from a personally meaningful prayer, or perhaps a name of God, whatever that means for you. If you are not religious, repeating a deeply felt one- or two-word virtue fulfills the same purpose: "compassion," "loving-kindness," or "justice" are three of many possibilities. A personal affirmation for healing can also serve as a mantra.

After a lot of practice in vocalizing the mantra during meditation—the amount of practice required is different for each person—the word has the power to create a specific thought pattern no matter your current situation. That means if you use this kind of meditation, eventually you can repeat the word to yourself wherever and whenever you desire and achieve the same calm, meditative feeling you get when meditating in a quiet place at home.

Beginners usually chant the mantra aloud, and some people use mala beads, a circular string of 108 beads akin to a rosary, to keep track of their progress while chanting. Both techniques create an external focus. The mala creates a tactile aspect to mantra meditation that can help the beginning meditator avoid becoming distracted by extraneous thoughts. Once you become experienced at this form of meditation, you can keep your focus internal by repeating the word silently and foregoing the mala.

To get a sense of how mantra meditation works, you can try it by repeating the word "love." Sit comfortably in a cross-legged position. Repeat the word ten times in a steady, even beat. Let this help you settle into the meditation. Then repeat it again, this time extending the vowel sound. Inhale, and say, "loooooooove." Let it last a few seconds, or as long as is comfortable for you. Find something for your mind to concentrate on. If you feel a vibration, perhaps in your chest, throat, or nose, you could attend to that. Or you could try bringing your awareness to your heart area. Notice if you feel a sensation there, perhaps a slight fullness or warmth. (It's also possible to feel a blockage there, especially if you are having a lot of difficulty with a relationship right now.) Another option is to create an image in your mind that goes along with the mantra, in this case perhaps a heart shape or an image of someone who embodies the word to you. If you think you might like this type of meditation but the word "love" is not working for you, you can try any other word; popular choices include "sun," "peace," or "God."

4. Prayer and Devotion

Prayer is about a conversation between a person and their higher power, whatever that means to each individual. Using prayer as a meditation is about communicating—talking and listening—with your conception of divinity (whether that's a divine being or nature) with an emphasis on listening. The person who meditates this way is in a receptive state of mind. The prayer is spoken, and then instead of repeating it like a mantra or moving on to something else, you stay with it. For example, after saying a prayer of thanks, you might dwell on thoughts of gratitude. Or you might simply wait in a state of appreciative patience. This receptive waiting is what makes prayer a meditative experience. It's important to note that like with affirmations, prayers for material benefits (e.g., a new car, a win for your sports team) don't create this kind of experience. Prayer of this kind is most effective when it is about relationships or rapport between the divine and the person praying.

Prayers for healing can be another form of meditation. One person or perhaps a group of people state a wish for another person to be healed in some way. Together they sit with that thought, imagining the object of their prayer. A common practice is to visualize the person surrounded by a light that emanates from the hearts of the people praying. Sitting quietly in contemplation is what makes this a form of meditation. Because it is done in relationship to another person (not staying internal to the meditator), it falls into the meditative prayer category.

Devoting your mind to nature is another way of moving beyond your everyday self and connecting with a higher reality, whether or not you believe that reality is divine. Understood this way, outdoor hikes, camping trips, or even a day at the beach provide opportunities for spiritual, meditative experiences. One way to engage in this form is to concentrate on one particular aspect of nature. The bubbling sound of a stream or the roar of ocean waves can create a profound internal experience. You might attach the sensation to a positive value, such as the receptiveness of the water or its power in the form of waves and tides. Lessons from nature abound. For example, noting how trees change with the seasons can be a lesson in accepting the inevitable changes in our personal lives and in society and the world around us. Or consider nature's uplifting reminder that connections exist among us all. The air that you exhale is inhaled by the plants around you and vice versa, in a never-ending cycle. The trees that provide shade for your street create homes for birds and squirrels. The clouds create the rain that provides water for trees, animals, and humans alike.

5. Contemplative Inquiry

This meditation path is the simplest to explain but for most people the hardest to do. The practice is to focus all our attention on one idea, so that the mind gravitates toward one single point. It's known as the intellectual's form of meditation, but the practice is difficult for them too. In general, well-educated people might be accustomed to focusing on a *complex* idea that gives the mind different thoughts to chew on, but the idea used here must necessarily be simple. One example is to concentrate on the idea of emptiness. To try this, sit quietly. Imagine all stimulation and stresses exiting your body, leaving you with a peaceful feeling of emptiness. Concentrate on the peaceful, empty state throughout your body, inhaling and exhaling the concept of empty space.

In Zen Buddhism, the use of the *koan*, or statement meant for contemplative inquiry, is another example of a concept for developing insight. One of the most well-known of these is: "What is the sound of one hand clapping?" Buddhist masters would ask monks and students this and similar questions as a way to monitor their progress and understanding of Buddhism's principles. A more modern application is to meditate on the large questions of humankind: Does God exist? Why is there suffering? These questions have many answers and at the same time no ultimate answer. They can be approached academically, studying the subjects, reading and learning what other minds have said, but that's a different undertaking. The goal of meditation is to let go of this type of complex thinking and take a simple—and therefore often more difficult—approach instead.

6. Mindfulness

Of the six types of meditation covered in this chapter, five are centered on *concentration*—on the breath, an image, a mantra, a relationship with the divine, or a concept. Mindfulness uses concentration also but then pairs it with *awareness*. While the first five ask the meditator to turn inward, mindfulness asks its practitioners to tune in inwardly and outwardly at the same time.

People who study mindfulness meditation often start by learning to notice their bodies in a new way. Like in other forms, first they observe their breath. Beyond that, mindfulness meditators ask questions such as, "How is my posture over the course of the day? How do pleasant or unpleasant events affect how I carry my body? What causes me to become tense, and where do I hold that tension in my body? Are there areas where my flow of blood or energy is constricted?" This practice develops new levels of awareness and also teaches practitioners a great deal about physical responses to everyday life events; observations that can be used to reduce tension and stress, thereby improving health.

The next step is to apply these same observational skills to our reactions to the world outside of us and to our own thoughts within. The goal is neutral and unemotional observation—that is, observation without the attachment of our usual personal or cultural judgments, expectations, or assumptions—and without the application the stories we unconsciously tell ourselves. Put another way, we cultivate what is called "the witness state" through mindfulness. This way of being allows you to be fully present in the moment and see what IS, without all your usual filters. On a practical level, the witness state affords a small bit of time and space between you and the outside world. It allows you the power to think before you respond to any given situation instead of reacting reflexively. And on a more spiritual level, it increases your awareness of the interconnections among all things—including yourself. You start to understand that you are not a separate or isolated being, but part of the greater whole.

To see how this can work on a basic level, the next time you eat a meal, try to describe it in terms of your senses instead of judgments. Opinions such as "this salad looks great" or "seems very fresh" or "is really big" are all judgments. Mindful descriptions would be, "There are many different vegetables and some nuts in this salad," "the colors are vibrant," "the salad fills this bowl entirely."

To see how this applies to people's behavior, imagine your boss walking toward you looking stressed. As a non-neutral, emotional response, your body would tense up but you wouldn't be aware of it. Your mind might think, "Here we go! She's going to project her stress and disrupt the office again because the report is late, but I was the only one of the team who did any work on it! But it seems like she's heading *my* way." A mindfully aware response would look something like: "My muscles are tensing and my throat feels full. My mind is making assumptions about what she's going to say." In the space of the witness state, you can gain mastery over yourself and decide how you want to respond. "I'm going to keep breathing and calm my body until I hear what she has to say. Then I will continue to breathe and stay calm while I consider her comments." With mindfulness meditation, you have the superpower of being able to remain calm, cool, and collected in the face of stresses large and small. This is different from suppressing your feelings or staying upbeat in all situations. It allows you to become aware of your emotional responses and respond appropriately, instead of being at their mercy.

The consequences of changing your thinking this way has profound potential. When you believe that your thoughts are the truth—as most of us do—it makes you not only pre-judge others but also limits your beliefs about yourself. Often people think they can't do something only to find the obstacles were all in their head. Mindfulness allows you to see your thoughts for what they are—ideas that you can choose to hold on to or choose to let go. From this type of clarity, freedom flows.

EXERCISE Choosing Your Method of Meditation

Part 2 of this exercise relates to aligning your natural tendencies with the six main types of meditation.

Set aside some time over the next week or two to explore the forms of meditation that resonated most with you. Try each of them a few times so you get a feel for them. After experimenting with those you resonated most with, perhaps try a couple other forms for a couple of days to see how they work for you in practice. Journal about your experiences as you practice. Include what you enjoy about the practice and write about the challenges you encounter. Keep an open, curious mind as you explore and remember that, as with any new skill, meditation takes time and practice to master. Be patient with yourself.

Following this exploration, we recommend continuing to practice the meditation form that works best for you to achieve a quieter mind and healthier life. Seek out groups that teach your preferred method and benefit from their refined teachings.

Tips for Overcoming Obstacles to Meditation Practice

While many well-intentioned people embark on a meditation practice, a good number find it challenging to maintain. For many of us, our days are filled to the brim with work, family, and community responsibilities. This simple fact is probably the most prevalent reason why people stop meditating. Meditating requires the commitment, flexibility, and quite possibly sacrifice of something else, to carve out at least twenty minutes a day on a regular basis. Before you begin meditating, make sure your expectations of yourself are clear and reasonable. Keeping an open mind sets the stage for a lasting practice.

Along with making time in the day for meditation, choosing a good time in life to initiate your practice can be an issue. It's understandable that someone would be motivated to start meditating at a very stressful time, but that's not often the best time to muster the resolve to take on a new practice that requires time and dedication. And again, you might just not be ready to meditate. Our brains can't go from super active or super anxious to cool, calm, and collected all at once. Just like an airplane slowing down along a runway, time and space are needed to decelerate. If you are under extreme stress and don't meditate, start with relaxation. Try reviewing the activities in this chapter and choose one to try daily.

Also remember that in the comprehensive model of health, all areas of our lives affect the others. Health arises from a synergy of positive choices. It doesn't require perfection, but it does need well-rounded effort to improve. We might want the benefits of meditation, but ingesting a lot of caffeine or sugar, not exercising, or making a habit of stoking negative emotions are all potential obstacles to sustaining a meditation practice.

When you are ready to start, remember that of the six different types, there are countless variations within each one. If you have trouble with one, that doesn't mean you have to give up on meditation altogether; another type may be the right choice for you. Joining a meditation group, where you can ask advice from fellow meditators and/or a group leader, can be very supportive.

Earlier we mentioned the varying claims about meditation, such as that it will make you more successful or help you lose weight. If you start to meditate with a specific outcome in mind, you could be disappointed. Meditation is a journey without a map. There is no doubt you will travel, but the odds of ending up in the same location as someone else are low, whether they are a friend, your yoga teacher, or a famous person you admire. The journey even varies for individual meditators day by day. On some days you may have a profound experience, on others you simply feel calmer, and on some particularly restless days, maybe not even that. Approached with an open mind, meditation is always a worthwhile journey.

One last thing: while the journey is worthwhile, that doesn't mean it will always be easy or even pleasant. Sometimes quieting the mind from our daily frenzy can give unwelcome thoughts a chance to rise to the surface. Though it's not often discussed in this way, meditation can bring us face to face with repressed memories and buried emotions that we haven't dealt with before. If we aren't prepared, it can be a difficult experience and stop a meditation practice in its tracks. If this is your situation, your first task will be to accept this difficult fact. Enlist the support of a therapist if necessary to assist with the exposed wounds. Follow your instincts about whether you want to continue meditating at this time, or if you need to pause and come back to it another time. Many people give up at this point, but there is good reason to continue when you can. The process may sometimes be painful, but the promise of healing awaits on the other side.

EXERCISE Your Personalized Plan for Developing
a Meditation Practice

Now that you have been introduced to the different forms of meditation and taken the opportunity to explore them, it's time to see how you can build meditation into your regular self-care routine. For this exercise, use the transformational steps Listen, Learn, Love, and Live to develop your practice goals. Use your journal to write out your plan.

Listen

Throughout this chapter, you have explored relaxation tools and the six forms of meditation. To establish your next steps, take a look at where you are currently in your meditation practice.

Do you currently have a regular or semi-regular meditation practice established?

- If yes:
  - How often do you meditate and for how long?
  - What do you have in place (personal strengths, resources, etc.) to support your current practice?
  - What barriers or challenges, both internal and external, inhibit your practice?
  - How would you like to see your practice evolve?
- If no:
  - What barriers prevent you from developing a regular meditation practice? List everything you can think of, both internal and external.
  - What strengths and resources are available to you that could support your practice?

Remember to approach this exercise with an open mind. Refrain from self-judgment.

Learn

Take out your journal and review your experiences from your exploration of the practices throughout this chapter. Consider both the relaxation tools and the meditation styles you learned here, as well as practices you've engaged in previously.

- Which practices came to you more easily?
- Were there some that you really enjoyed but found more challenging? What was challenging about them?
- Which practices did you resonate with most (regardless of the level of ease)?
- As you consider incorporating meditation into your routine, what challenges do you foresee?
  - What are some ways that you can reduce or eliminate some of the identified challenges?
- What strengths and resources are available to support your new or expanded meditation practice? Be creative.

Based on your reflection, choose one or two practices to incorporate into your personalized self-care routine.

Love

Begin practicing daily, if possible, or at least several times a week. If your lifestyle allows, it is recommended that you identify a set time each day that is dedicated to your meditation practice. For those who have jobs or other circumstances that create an inconsistent schedule, work your meditation time in where it best fits each day. Put it into your calendar.

Be patient with yourself, especially if you have never or rarely meditated before. Just as you would not expect to master the piano the first time you play, it takes time to develop the skill of quieting your mind.

As you practice, continue to observe and journal about your experiences. Notice the changes that you experience on each level of the koshas: body, energy, mind, intellect, and spirit.

Live

Continue to build your meditation practice as part of your lifestyle. Once you have a routine established, you may choose different forms of meditation to learn over time. For example, you may choose to spend a few months focusing on breath meditation, and then spend the next few months working with mantras, and so forth.

Chapter Summary

Relaxation and deep breathing exercises are helpful precursors to meditation. The goal of meditation is to cultivate self-understanding about how you perceive life and your thoughts. A clear mind from meditative exercise leads to healthy life decisions. The six ways to meditate are breath, visualization and affirmation, mantra, prayer, contemplation, and mindfulness. Find the one that suits you and go with that method. The first five meditation methods are concentration-based while Mindfulness is awareness-based. Start slowly with relaxation and meditation practices and patiently build a habit into your routine.

Meditation brings health to a new level. It opens doors inward into ourselves, introducing us to new opportunities for insight, for clearing out the hurts and wounds that all of us accumulate as we live in the world. Your path to meditation will be unpredictable, uniquely yours. It is a path toward peace.

In the next and final chapter on spirituality and health, you will uncover the healing power of your connection to nature and/or your higher power.

Twelve
TAPPING INTO SPIRITUALITY

Terms such as "spirituality," "faith," "higher power," and other religion-related words often conjure thoughts of the other-worldly and unknowable aspects of life. In a pluralistic society where some people believe in their personal religion, others are atheists and others follow non-traditional paths, remaining inclusive to each reader is a challenge—so please read this chapter with the idea that larger spiritual beliefs exist in every healing tradition in the world. The beliefs are very hard to prove and even harder to discuss in a simple chapter like this. Just know that your deeper spiritual beliefs are present in every part of the world, simply in different forms.

In this chapter, spirituality is also compatible with any form of religion or spirituality you might already practice, including non-belief. Recall from chapter 2, the bhakti path of yoga asks us to draw on the spiritual beliefs and practices that uplift our sense of being and bring us into connection with something greater than ourselves. The intention of this chapter is to help you think about what spirituality means for you, then help you harness that spirituality to motivate you toward achieving your highest health goals.

We'll guide you in identifying what is spiritual for you, then explore how to harness that spirituality to help you attain your health goals. You will learn how to apply yoga practices to spirituality and have an opportunity to create a personal plan for integrating spirituality into your whole health lifestyle.

Spirituality and Science

Health and spirituality may strike you as a strange pairing, but that wasn't always the case. From ancient times to the early 1900s, medicine and healing were enmeshed with medicine and spirituality. For most of that time there was no perceived division between body, mind, and spirit. "Healthy" meant the health of all three, and illness affected them all together.

Following the scientific advances of the late 1800s and early 1900s, medicine and healing shifted away from spirit to concentrate more and more exclusively on physical health. In 1910, an influential report about medical education in the United States and Canada, conducted by the Carnegie Foundation, proclaimed that medicine was a strictly scientific affair, within which was no room for religion.[52]

For decades, medicine advanced in that direction, with astounding results. But the pendulum began the swing back by a small amount in the 1960s and '70s toward a more balanced view. Today, that movement continues. The connection between mind and body is more widely accepted. Complementary and alternative forms of healing are making their way into some of our most high-tech hospitals.

Spirituality in Action

With a goal of respecting each belief system, in yoga therapy circles spirituality is defined in terms of the higher self: the wise and unchanging being that exists for all of us. We are in touch with that self when we feel at our best, when we feel most like our true selves. That feeling might be brought out during an activity people usually associate with spirituality, such as prayer, meditation, walking in nature; or a hobby, like gardening, drawing, or singing. For some people, it happens when they are working toward an ideal such

---

52. Christina Maria Puchalski, "Religion, Medicine and Spirituality: What We Know, What We Don't Know and What We Do," *Asian Pacific Journal of Cancer Prevention* 11, 2010, supplement 1:45–49. https://www.ncbi.nlm.nih.gov/pubmed/20590349.

as charity, beauty, or justice in their professional or personal lives. Sometimes people access that higher self during unplanned peak moments when the circumstances are just right—hearing the laughter of children or viewing a ray of sunlight through clouds. Take some time to reflect on what elicits these kinds of spiritual senses in you.

EXERCISE Connecting to Your Higher Self Through Joy

Through the experience of joy, you create a "fast-track" to connection with your higher self. In this exercise, you will explore your pathways to joy. Take out your journal, begin thinking back to different times in your life when you experienced joy.

As a young child, what were your favorite activities and games? Did you like to tumble and roll your body? Play on a swing set or jungle gym? Chase butterflies? Create with clay, crayons, or finger paints? Play chase or tag with your friends? List as many activities you can think of. To help get more in touch with your younger self and have some fun with it, perhaps write or draw the activities with markers or crayons.

Continue this inquiry through different stages of your life, from early childhood through now. What brings you joy, makes you laugh, and gives you pleasure?

When you have finished, go back and review your list. Pick one or two activities that resonate with you and do them within the next week. Notice how you feel while you engage in the activity. Consider each of the layers: body, energy, mind, intellect, and spirit.

• • • • ● • • • •

Another way to become conscious of your spiritual experiences is to form statements of belief. These are the brief, true statements that we may or may not consciously recognize, but that drive us toward our own sense of purpose and meaning. They are the tenets that direct our lives. To help you think about your spirituality, view this wide-ranging list of beliefs that people hold. See which ones resonate with you.

• I love my family and friends.
• My belief in God is the center of my life.

- Health is wealth.
- Balanced nutrition is the key to a healthy life.
- Serving others brings freedom.
- Daily exercise is how I find peace of body and mind.
- Animals are an inspiration.
- Daily prayer and meditation are a key to my well-being.
- Lifelong learning is my source of happiness.
- Rest sustains my health.
- Living a sustainable life connects me to Mother Earth.
- Gardening brings me close to nature.
- Trees inspire me.
- When I grow and cook vegetables, I know that the earth cares for us.
- Pursuing justice is doing God's work.
- Making moral choices is the essence of being human.
- Striving for excellence shows the best of the human spirit.
- Beauty in art stirs my soul.
- Teaching children nourishes me.
- When I care for the ill, I know I'm doing what I'm meant to do.
- Singing makes me happy to my soul.
- God wants us to be joyful.
- I'm most myself when I'm dancing.
- Learning other people's stories connects us together as humans.
- Laughter is the best medicine.

EXERCISE Your Spiritual Beliefs

In this exercise, you continue to explore and reflect on your spiritual beliefs through creative expression. To begin, identify any of the previously listed beliefs that align with your core values and add any that are not listed. Then use your chosen creative form of expression to express those beliefs into form. Create a collage. Draw or paint a picture that represents your beliefs. Get some clay and mold a statue that depicts them. Write a poem or song.

Choreograph a dance. Have fun with it as you allow your spirit to move through you. It doesn't matter what level of artistic skill you have. The intention is simply to have fun as you explore and express your beliefs.

Remain mindful throughout the process, noticing how you are feeling in all layers.

After completing this exercise, you can use what you created as a reminder of your values in daily life.

• • • • ● • • • •

Hopefully the spiritual statements that speak to you reflect activities that are already primary in your life. If not, allow this exercise to inspire you to investigate how you might make more room for them. Other chapters have already mentioned devoting more time to hobbies, or friends, or making sure you get outdoors. Perhaps you even must think about changing to a different career. No one goes to a job interview and asks, "How will this job connect me to my higher power?" But finding meaning in work enriches our lives, while working without meaning can yield emptiness.

Additional journaling or talking with a trusted confidante may help you move further along in this process. Talking about spirituality is more comfortable for some of us than others. Unless you belong to a religious or spiritual community, it is not the kind of thing that is usually discussed, and if you do belong but are questioning aspects of that community, it may not feel acceptable to share your thoughts with its members. Professional therapists or spiritual counselors may be of assistance. Since yoga therapy works at the intersection of spirit, body, and mind, a yoga therapist is very well-suited as a guide for this type of exploration.

Health and Your Spiritual Values

Making healthful changes requires time, effort, and the ability to persevere through challenges. Knowing that something is "good for us" in the long run does not always mean we're going to find the motivation to do it.[53] Tapping

---

53. As cited in, for example, Kacey Ballard and Brian Knutson, "Dissociable Neural Representations of Future Reward Magnitude and Delay During Temporal Discounting," *Neuroimage* 45 (1): 143–150. Mar 1, 2009. Published online November 2008. DOI: 10.1016/j.neuroimage .2008.11.004.

into spiritual values can help you overcome the temptation of short-term rewards that interfere with our long-term goals. For some, spiritual values are related to feelings of happiness and freedom; for others, they can help to foster discipline. A commitment to justice can motivate an activist to work for a valued cause diligently over time. The discipline of religious observance may be transferred from the spiritual arena of life to the physical. The key is to identify values that have meaning for you in your life right now. For example, if a primary value for you is relationships, think about how improving your lifestyle will benefit your family. Maybe you'll have the energy to help your daughter practice her soccer skills, or your spouse will worry less about your health. Alternately, perhaps health is one of your highest values but it's hard for you to find time for relationships. Reading about how strong relationships benefit physical health may motivate you to find a better balance. In another instance, if an underlying value is the pursuit of excellence in a field, then improving your health will make you better able to achieve it.

Less pleasant emotions can make effective motivators but are detrimental to comprehensive health. Fear may spur us into action but it is triggered by the fight or flight response, and as we've discussed, spending too much time in this state erodes our health over time. Jealousy or revenge can direct us but also harm our spirits as well as our bodies. Spiritual motivation lets us achieve our comprehensive health goals to benefit body, mind, and spirit all as one. The stories below of Christie and John exemplify what we mean.

Christie was a busy, successful executive with a prestigious and high-paying job, but it was very stressful. Just a few years into her career, she was already starting to feel burned out. Christie loved the job, but it was all-consuming. She felt like it was all she had, and she found it just wasn't enough. To make matters worse, overeating unhealthy food was one of her favorite forms of solace. Christie wasn't depressed, but she was worried she was heading in that direction.

Christie could sometimes get to yoga class and decided to sign on for yoga therapy with one of her favorite teachers. Her stated goal for yoga therapy was to lose fifteen pounds. But she and the yoga therapist quickly deduced that there was a deeper problem: life was just no fun anymore. Christie had lost her spirit, her zest. She realized she was missing a sense of freedom, one that she used to find especially when she was outdoors. She smiled as she remembered that when she was a kid, her dad nicknamed her "Natural C," because she loved nature so much. So Christie set a goal, instead, to recapture Natural C.

Every first weekend of the month, Christie made time to hike through the woods. She was surprised at how quickly her Natural C spirit began to return. The next month, Christie continued her hikes and set about redecorating her office to bring the outdoors in. She added plants, wooden accent pieces, and nature photographs. At times, she played nature sounds on low volume. The third month, she extended the theme to nutrition by eating only natural foods. Losing weight became a by-product of reclaiming her spirit. Now Christie was back to her full self, an adult version of Natural C who could handle her work stress and be happy.

For Christie, spirituality meant feelings of happiness and freedom. For others, spirituality can help to foster discipline. A passion for exercise might motivate a long-distance runner to practice every day, in all kinds of weather. It worked something like that for John:

John was frustrated and, if he was honest with himself, a bit defeated. He had two great reasons to stay healthy. His father was just diagnosed with diabetes, so John knew that he could easily face the same future if he didn't learn to take better care of himself. Plus, his long-term relationship had just ended, and he thought a leaner body would help him feel more confident about dating. But John struggled to stick to any kind of fitness program or healthy diet. Sometimes he would go all in at a gym for a few weeks but then overdo it and have to stop. Sometimes he ate well, but the process was slow and he found junk food very hard to resist. Even though he knew it wasn't true, in some moments a healthy lifestyle just didn't seem worth the effort. Every night he prayed for the health and happiness of his loved ones and himself. He sat in meditative silence.

When John happened to mention his journey about diet and exercise to his pastor, his pastor suggested that John use his religious devotion to help him lead a healthy lifestyle. He explained: "Think of exercise as a way to thank God for the body you were given. The gym could be like your second temple And healthy food is also God's gift to you. Eat only the natural foods that were divinely created." He tried the yoga class to help him connect his mind and body with his spirit. The prescription worked. Viewed in this way, it was easy for John to find the discipline to exercise and eat healthily. He knew he was preserving his body for the long haul, increasing the odds that it would stay healthy. Aligning his religious beliefs with his physical health worked for John.

Health, Spirituality, and Healing

Spirituality can aid with healing, but in some cases, spiritual difficulties are things people need to heal from. Can you relate? Many people today feel internally conflicted by religion and spirituality. We may crave the comfort, spirituality, and camaraderie of religious communities we grew up in. But some of us may be uncomfortable with beliefs that originate from a time in history when cultural norms were far from what we find acceptable now. Some may have had negative experiences with members of the community or with spiritual leaders, ranging from small to traumatic incidents with emotional scarring as the result.

Being alienated from a childhood religion or witnessing tragedy and suffering that religion can't adequately explain can leave some people angry, confused, and feeling divided from their sense of spirituality. This can lead to a sense of isolation or abandonment, which all too often lead to compounding the issues associated with negative health choices.

These sorts of wounds are difficult to heal. Putting religious teachings into historical perspective can be one way to see the issues in a different light. Finding other like-minded people lends support and empathy for our ways of thinking. Seeking counseling, whether from a therapist or clergy person, can help us to process emotions so they no longer get in our way. Other approaches can be found in other chapters of this book. Since religion is ultimately about relationship, reviewing that chapter may offer tools to help solve or relieve the problem. The meditation chapter, particularly the section on meditation through prayer or devotion, offers practices that may kindle your insight.

Spirituality and Comprehensive Health

Look back at your list of spiritual belief statements from earlier in this chapter and think about the ones you chose. You'll probably notice that many of the beliefs relate back to other health areas in this book. Some of the spiritual beliefs listed refer to fitness, nutrition, or rest. Some relate to work, the environment, or relationships. Some are about hobbies or prayer and meditation. As covered in the section on finance, you may be wealthy in your spiritual piggy bank. All of the chapters, then, come full circle in the wheel of life and health.

EXERCISE Your Personalized Plan for Tapping Into Spirituality

Throughout this chapter, you have explored spirituality, connected with your higher self through joyful experiences, and used creativity to express your core values. Next, you'll create your personalized plan for expanding your spiritual practice. Use your journal to write out your plan.

Listen

Think about your spiritual values, current activities that connect you with your higher self, and other spiritual practices that are already part of your routine. Make a list if that helps you focus. As you reflect, consider the following:

- How do you feel when engaged in these practices?
    - Do they truly connect you to your higher self?
    - Are the practices uplifting?
    - Do you feel resistance around any of them?
    - Are these practices that you purposefully chose or that you do because of expectations given by others?
- List the practices that are most fulfilling to you.
- Are there other practices that you would like to explore (from this book or other sources)?
- Do you strive to live according to the values that you identified?
    - Some may be easier than others. Make note of which are easy for you as well as those you find challenging.
    - List ways in which you actively live your values.
- What supports your spiritual connection and practice routines?
- List any challenges that hinder your practice.

Use this inquiry to identify where you are and your intentions for moving forward.

Learn

Using the information you've gained from this book, your experiences as you explored the previous exercises, and the insights you received in your Listen inquiry, what is your goal for expanding your spiritual practice? Take some time to discern where you want to grow and how to get there.

- What shifts do you want to make in your spiritual practice?
- How do you see these changes impacting your health and well-being?
- What resources do you need to empower yourself to succeed?
- What challenges do you foresee?
    - How can you mitigate those challenges?
- Identify your motivation.

As you create your plan to implement the changes you wish to create, consider the individual steps along the way. Include strategies for harnessing your resources and overcoming challenges.

Love

Choose a starting point to implement your plan. If you have multiple changes you want to make, consider starting with one and working the others in over time. Start implementing the new practice over the next few weeks. Remain mindful, taking note of how you are feeling and what changes you are making. Be aware of your thoughts (both supportive and not) and how they influence your practice. Evaluate the results of the practices. Are they bringing the results you seek? Make changes and adjustments where needed. Once you feel solid in the new practice, then choose the next practice that you wish to explore.

Live

Continue your spiritual practices so that they become an integrated part of your self-care routine. Remain mindful of how you feel as you practice, and aware of how your practice affects your life. Make adjustments where needed.

Chapter Summary

In this chapter, you explored the role of spiritual connection in health and well-being and learned how clear, reasonable and engaged spiritual beliefs reduce stress by presenting a larger picture and an acceptance of the unexplainable aspects of life. The scientific community is beginning to recognize the importance of the mind-body connection in health care. Studies show that a healthy spiritual connection has a positive impact on health, while rigid and dogmatic belief systems have an increased prevalence of depression and poor health. Research shows that practicing gratitude and experiencing joy bring an increased sense of satisfaction in life.

The practices of yoga aim to harness one's existing beliefs for positive healthy behaviors. The Comprehensive Yoga therapy model interprets spirituality as fostering a strong connection with your higher self. Finding peace with the religious perspective you inherited as a child can free up motivation for your present. Your spiritual values can motivate you, foster discipline, and lead to greater happiness and improved health.

conclusion
WHAT'S NEXT?

Usually when you come to the end of a book, you are finished. In this case, making yourself fully healthy is a daily endeavor. There is always more to do. We invite you to continue working with this book. Select the lifestyle areas that spoke the most to you, perhaps the ones touched on by your spiritual belief statements; or others if they seem more pressing or more relevant to your experience. Read those chapters again, then use the information to plan and make further changes. Set specific goals and track your progress. Keep them finite and realistic, to make sure you can meet them. You'll make more progress in the long run by setting and achieving small goals, than by aiming for huge changes and getting discouraged. Continue to reflect. Write in a journal. Consider invoking the assistance of professionals.

Remember, yoga philosophy tells us that we are five beings: spiritual, physical, energetic, emotional, and intellectual, all at the same time. By attending to your full comprehensive self, you can ensure yourself the healthiest possible life.

ACKNOWLEDGMENTS

From Bob Butera

I dedicate this book to all the people who use this knowledge for their personal health and well-being. To all the teachers in the world who use this and other information to inspire and guide others on their healing journey, I salute you.

When I reached The Yoga Institute of Mumbai, India, all the pieces of my searching were represented in one place. The physical, emotional, relational, attitude of work, nutrition, exercise, and spiritual practice and the integrated perspective in which they are taught there completed my search. I have deep appreciation for my primary teachers, Dr. Jayadeva and Hansaji Yogendra, Mrs. Armaiti Desai, Harry and Promil Sequeira, and all of those who support, uplift and disseminate the teachings of The Yoga Institute around the world.

The staff, teachers, and students at the YogaLife Institute over the last 25+ years have offered much support, insight and dedication to the field of Yoga. The work that they do keeps YogaLife a thriving hub of consciousness and transformation, and I am eternally grateful for all of their efforts, large and small.

The instructors and graduates of our Comprehensive Yoga therapy training over the years helped our message be tested and continually refined. Jennifer Kreatsoulas and Erika Tenenbaum have been tremendous leaders and examples of the yoga lifestyle. Staffan Elgelid has consistently supported the program, as has co-founder Erin Byron, who passionately teaches Yoga therapy. It is a blessing to see all of the amazing contributions they are making to the world.

We honor our friends and colleagues at the International Association of Yoga Therapists for their hard work and dedication to the field.

My professors at the Earlham School of Religion, especially Ann Miller and Alan Kolp, who recommended I make "Yoga therapy" my ministry. And, to the professors at the California Institute of Integral Studies, namely Dr. Jim Ryan and Dr. Yi Wu for their wisdom and guidance during my Yoga therapy PhD, and Dr. Eleanor Criswell for her support.

Of course, no acknowledgment would be complete without recognizing my wife, Kristen. She is my partner on the path of enlightenment, who supports and uplifts me in more ways than I could possibly list here. Your love is a gift that knows no end—thank you for it all.

From Ilene Rosen

This book is for all of the teachers in my life. To my yoga teachers in the Comprehensive Yoga therapy program at YogaLife Institute, the learning you communicated continues to astound. To my yoga teacher training teachers at Yoga on Main and Yoga Child in Philadelphia, for showing me how broadly and deeply yoga reaches and where to find the fun in it.

To all my parents and grandparents, who taught me just about everything I need in life, and who believed I could write a book. To my schoolteachers over the years and my editors at Scholastic, Inc., who built and shaped my writing.

Most of all, to my husband, Mark Rosen, and my daughters, Pamela, Caroline, and Julia. It's all for you.

From Jennifer Hilbert

I would like to thank the whole YogaLife community including Kristen Butera, Erin Byron, and Staffan Elgelid for facilitating and fostering this amazing incubator of learning and exploration … what a gift!

I would like to thank all of the yoga therapy students I have mentored and taught and all of my clients. I hope you have learned as much from me as I have from you. You all continue to inspire me.

I would like to thank my friends and family, especially Josh, Sam, and Amelia for supporting and encouraging me. Love you all dearly.

BIBLIOGRAPHY

Bond, Annie B. *Home Enlightenment: Create a Nurturing, Healthy, and Toxin-Free Home.* New York: Rodale, 2005.

Butera, Robert. *Meditation for Your Life: Creating a Plan that Suits Your Style.* Woodbury, MN: Llewellyn Worldwide, 2012.

———. *The Pure Heart of Yoga: Ten Essential Steps for Personal Transformation.* Woodbury, MN: Llewellyn Worldwide, 2009.

Butera, Robert, Erin Byron, and Staffan Elgelid. *Yoga Therapy for Stress and Anxiety: Create a Personalized Holistic Plan to Balance Your Life.* Woodbury, MN: Llewellyn Worldwide, 2015

Butera, Robert, and Jennifer Kreatsoulas. *Body Mindful Yoga: Create a Powerful and Affirming Relationship with Your Body.* Woodbury, MN: Llewellyn Worldwide, 2018

Butera, Kristen, and Staffan Elgelid. *Yoga Therapy: A Personalized Approach for Your Active Lifestyle.* Champaign, IL: Human Kinetics, 2017.

Chödrön, Pema. *When Things Fall Apart.* Boston: Shambhala Publications, 1997.

Easwaran, Ecknath (translator). *Bhagavad Gita.* Berkeley: New Mountain Center of Meditation, 2007.

———. *The Upanishads.* Berkeley: New Mountain Center of Meditation, 2007.

Eifert, Georg, and John P. Forsyth. *The Mindfulness and Acceptance Workbook for Anxiety.* Oakland, CA: New Harbinger, 2008.

Eisenstein, Charles. *The Yoga of Eating: Transcending Diets and Dogma to Nourish the Natural Self.* Washington, D.C.: New Trends Publishing, 2003.

Emerson, David, and Elizabeth Hopper. *Overcoming Trauma through Yoga.* Berkeley: North Atlantic Books, 2011.

Feuerstein, Georg. *The Shambhala Encyclopedia of Yoga.* Boston: Shambhala Publications, 1997.

Forbes, Bo. *Yoga for Emotional Balance: Simple Practices to Help Relieve Anxiety and Depression.* Boston: Shambhala, 2011.

Govindan, Marshall. *Kriya Yoga Sutras of Patanjali and the Siddhas.* Quebec: Kriya Yoga Publications, 2001.

Greenberger, Dennis, and Christine A. Padesky. *Mind Over Mood.* New York: Guilford Press, 1995.

Herrigel, Eugen. *Zen in the Art of Archery.* New York: Pantheon Books, 1953.

Horowitz, Ellen G., and Staffan Elgelid. *Yoga Therapy: Theory and Practice.* London: Routledge, 2015.

James, William. *The Varieties of Religious Experience.* Originally published 1902 by Longmans, Green & Co., London. Reprinted 1985 by Penguin Classics, New York.

Judith, Anodea. *Wheels of Life: A User's Guide to the Chakra System.* St. Paul, MN: Llewellyn Worldwide, 1999.

Kataria, Madan. *Laughter Yoga: Daily Practices for Health and Happiness.* New York: Penguin Books, 2018.

Keleman, Stanley. *Emotional Anatomy: The Structure of Experience.* Westlake Village, UK: Center Press, 1989.

Li, Qing. *Forest Bathing: How Trees Can Help You Find Health and Happiness.* New York: Viking Press, 2018.

Louv, Richard. *The Nature Principle: Reconnecting with Life in a Virtual Age.* Chapel Hill, NC: Algonquin Books, 2011.

Newcomb, Sarah, *Loaded: Money, Psychology, and How to Get Ahead Without Leaving Your Values Behind.* Hoboken, NJ: Wiley, 2016.

Quach, Due, *Calm Clarity: How to Use Science to Rewire Your Brain for Greater Wisdom, Fulfillment, and Joy.* New York: TarcherPerigree/Random House, 2018.

Shri Yogendra. *Guide to Yoga Meditation.* Mumbai: The Yoga Institute Press, 1983.

———. *Yoga Cyclopedia I for Yoga Postures.* Mumbai: The Yoga Institute Press, 1982.

Swami Muktibodhana. *Hatha Yoga Pradipika.* Bihar: Bihar School of Yoga Pub., 1998.

Swami Rama, Rudolph Ballentine, and Alan Hymes. *Science of Breath: A Practical Guide.* Honesdale, PA: The Himalayan Institute Press, 1998.

Swami Vivekananda. *Karma-Yoga and Bhakti-Yoga.* Buckinghamshire, UK: Ramakrishna Vedanta Centre, 1980.

To Write to the Authors

If you wish to contact the author or would like more information about this book, please write to the author in care of Llewellyn Worldwide Ltd. and we will forward your request. Both the author and publisher appreciate hearing from you and learning of your enjoyment of this book and how it has helped you. Llewellyn Worldwide Ltd. cannot guarantee that every letter written to the author can be answered, but all will be forwarded. Please write to:

Robert Butera, PhD
Ilene S. Rosen
Jennifer Hilbert
℅ Llewellyn Worldwide
2143 Wooddale Drive
Woodbury, MN 55125-2989
Please enclose a self-addressed stamped envelope for reply,
or $1.00 to cover costs. If outside the U.S.A., enclose
an international postal reply coupon.

Many of Llewellyn's authors have websites with additional
information and resources. For more information,
please visit our website at http://www.llewellyn.com